CARDIOMYOPLASTY

The Bakken Research Center Series
Volume 3

edited by:

Alain Carpentier, M.D., Ph.D.
Professor, Université de Paris VI
Chief, Department of Cardiovascular Surgery
Hôpital Broussais
Paris, France

Juan-Carlos Chachques, M.D.
Department of Cardiovascular Surgery
Hôpital Broussais
Paris, France

Pierre A. Grandjean, M.S.
Bakken Research Center
Maastricht, The Netherlands

**Futura Publishing
Company, Inc.**
Mount Kisco, NY
1991

Library of Congress Cataloging-in-Publication Data

Cardiomyoplasty / edited by Alain Carpentier, Juan-Carlos Chachques,
   Pierre A. Grandjean.
       p.   cm. — (The Bakken Research Center series ; v. 3)
   Includes papers presented at the First International Meeting on
Cardiomyoplasty in Paris on June 1989.
   Includes bibliographical references and index.
   ISBN 0-87993-395-X
   1. Cardiomyoplasty—Congresses. I. Carpentier, Alain, M.D.
II. Chachques, Juan-Carlos. III. Grandjean, Pierre A.
IV. International Meeting on Cardiomyoplasty (1st : 1989 : Paris,
France) V. Series.
   [DNLM: 1. Heart Surgery—methods—congresses. 2. Muscles—
Transplantation—congresses. WG 169 C2678 1989]
   RD598.35.C37C37   1991
   617.4′120592—dc20
   DNLM/DLC
   for Library of Congress   91-6593
                                                                   CIP

Copyright © 1991
Futura Publishing Company, Inc.

Published by
Futura Publishing Company, Inc.
2 Bedford Ridge Road
Mount Kisco, New York 10549

L. C. No.: 91-6593
ISBN No.: 0-87993-395X

Every effort has been made to ensure that the information in this book is as
up to date and accurate as possible at the time of publication. However, due
to the constant developments in medicine, neither the author, nor the editor,
nor the publisher can accept any legal or any other responsibility for any errors
or omissions that may occur.

Printed in the United States of America

**To the Memory of
Professor Charles Dubost**

a great surgeon,
a great teacher,
a great man

Contributors

Bernard Abry, M.D. Intensive Care Specialist, Department of Cardiovascular Surgery, Hôpital Broussais, Paris, France

Christophe Acar, M.D. Assistant, Department of Cardiovascular Surgery, Hôpital Broussais, Paris, France

David R. Anderson, M.D. Research Associate, Division of Cardiothoracic Surgery, Wayne State University, Detroit, Michigan

Giorgio Arpesella, M.D. Cardiac Surgeon, Cattedra di Chirurgia del Cuore e Grossi Vasi, Ospendal S. Orsola, Univesita di Bologna, Bologna, Italy

Regent L. Beaudet, M.D. Chairman, Department of Cardiothoracic Surgery, Hôpital Notre-Dame, Montreal, Canada

Danielle Bensasson, M.D. Anesthesiologist, Department of Cardiovascular Surgery, Hôpital Broussais, Paris, France

Charles R. Bridges, Jr., M.D., Ph.D. Research Associate, Division of Cardiothoracic Surgery, University of Pennsylvania, Philadelphia, Pennsylvania

Alain Carpentier, M.D., Ph.D. Professor, University of Paris VI, Chief, Department of Cardiovascular Surgery, Hôpital Broussais, Paris, France

Ugo Carraro, M.D. Associate Professor of General Pathology, C.N.R. Unit for Muscle Biology and Physiopathology, Institute of General Pathology, University of Padova, Padova, Italy

Lon Castle, M.D. The Cleveland Clinic Foundation, Cleveland, Ohio

Juan-Carlos Chachques, M.D. Assistant, Cardiovascular Surgery, Department of Cardiovascular Surgery, Hôpital Broussais, Paris, France

Ray C-J. Chiu, M.D., Ph.D. Professor of Surgery, The Montreal General Hospital, McGill University, Montreal, Quebec, Canada

Ignacio Y. Christlieb, Ph.D. Director, Thoracic Surgery Research Laboratory, Allegheny Singer Research Institute, Allegheny Campus of the Medical College of Pennsylvania, Pittsburgh, Pennsylvania

Delos M. Cosgrove, M.D. Chairman, Department of Cardiothoracic Surgery, The Cleveland Clinic Foundation, Cleveland, Ohio

Jean Fissette, M.D. Professor of Anatomy, University Hospital of Liege Sart Tilman, Belgium

Jacques Fourny, M.D. Associate Professor, Cardiovascular Surgery, Department of Cardiovascular Surgery, University Hospital of Liege Sart Tilman, Belgium

Manfred Frey, M.D. Professor of Plastic Surgery, Division of Hand, Plastic and Reconstructive Surgery, Department of Surgery, Medical School of the University of Zurich, Zurich, Switzerland

Akira Furuse Department of Thoracic Surgery, University of Tokyo, Tokyo, Japan

Pierre A. Grandjean, M.S. Biomechanical Engineer, Bakken Research Center, Maastricht, The Netherlands

Helmut Gruber, M.D. Professor of Anatomy, Head of the Institute of Anatomy, University of Vienna, Vienna, Austria

Robert L. Hammond, B.S. Chief Technician, Division of Cardiothoracic Surgery, Wayne State University, Detroit, Michigan

W. Happak Second Surgical University Clinic, Vienna, Austria

J. Donald Hill, M.D. Chairman, Department of Cardiovascular Surgery, Pacific Presbyterian Medical Center, San Francisco, California

Jonathan C. Jarvis, B.Sc., Ph.D. University Research Fellow, Department of Human Anatomy and Cell Biology and Muscle Research Centre, University of Liverpool, Liverpool, United Kingdom

Adib D. Jatene, M.D. Heart Institute, Sao Paulo University Medical School, Sao Paulo, Brazil

Byron A. Kakulas, M.D. Professor and Head, Department of Neuropathology, Royal Perth Hospital, Neuromuscular Research Institute, University of West Australia, Perth, Australia

Race L. Kao, Ph.D. Professor and Director, Surgical Research, Allegheny Singer Research Institute, Allegheny Campus of the Medical College of Pennsylvania, Pittsburgh, Pennsylvania

Jean Philippe Kieffer, M.D. Intensive Care Specialist, Department of Cardiovascular Surgery, Hôpital Broussais, Paris, France

Carlos M. Li, M.D. Research Fellow, The Montreal General Hospital, McGill University, Montreal, Quebec, Canada

Raymond Limet, M.D. Professor of Surgery, Department of Cardiovascular Surgery, University Hospital of Liege Sart Tilman, Belgium

Didier Loulmet, M.D. Assistant, Cardiovascular Surgery, Department of Cardiovascular Surgery, Hôpital Broussais, Paris, France

Caroline M.H.B. Lucas, M.D. Resident Cardiology, Department of Cardiology, University Hospital Maastricht, University of Limburg, Maastricht, The Netherlands

George J. Magovern, M.D. Chairman and Professor, Department of Surgery, Allegheny General Hospital, Allegheny Campus of the Medical College of Pennsylvania, Pittsburgh, Pennsylvania

Serban Mihaileanu, M.D. Consultant in Cardiology, Department of Cardiovascular Surgery, Hôpital Broussais, Paris, France

Luiz Felipe P. Moreira, M.D. Heart Institute, Sao Paulo University Medical School, Sao Paulo, Brazil

Yoshihiro Naruse Department of Thoracic Surgery, University of Tokyo, Tokyo, Japan

Roberto Novoa, M.D. Staff Surgeon, The Cleveland Clinic Foundation, Cleveland, Ohio

Olaf C.K.M. Penn, M.D. Professor of Cardiothoracic Surgery, Department of Cardiac Surgery, University Hospital Maastricht, Maastricht, The Netherlands

Patrick Perier, M.D. Associate Professor, Cardiovascular Surgery, Department of Cardiovascular Surgery, Hôpital Broussais, Paris, France

Dirk Pette, M.D. Professeur de Biochimie et Chairman, Fakultät für Biologie, Universität Konstanz, Konstanz, Germany

Marc A. Radermecker, M.D. Assistant, Cardiovascular Surgery, University Hospital of Liege Sart Tilman, Belgium

Stanley Salmons, B.Sc., M.Sc., Ph.D. Professor of Medical Cell Biology, Department of Human Anatomy and Cell Biology and Muscle Research Centre, University of Liverpool, Liverpool, United Kingdom

Maria J.W. Smets, M.D. Staff Anesthesiologist, Department of Anesthesiology, University Hospital Maastricht, Maastricht, The Netherlands

Olav M. Sola, M.D. Senior Research Associate Professor, Department of Surgery, University of Washington, and Director of Cardiomyoplasty Research, The Hope Heart Institute, Seattle, Washington

Larry W. Stephenson, M.D. Professor of Surgery, Chief, Division of Cardiothoracic Surgery, Wayne State University, Detroit, Michigan

Tatsuhiko Takahama Department of Thoracic Surgery, University of Tokyo, Tokyo, Japan

Herwig Thoma, D. Techn Professor of Biomedical Technique and Physics, Head of the Bioengineering Laboratory, Second Surgical University Clinic Vienna, Austria

Robert Thomas, B.A. Research Technologist Supervisor, Division of Cardiothoracic Surgery, Department of Surgery, University of Washington, Seattle, Washington

FH Van Der Veen Academic Hospital Maastricht, Maastricht, The Netherlands

Foreword

The use of skeletal muscle to repair, reinforce, or replace the heart has been a dream for many years; a dream as old as Jesus and Christ! In 1931, F.R. Jesus, a Puerto Rican surgeon, was the first to replace a portion of the left ventricle with a skeletal muscle in a human being,[1] and in 1982, J.E. Christ, an English surgeon, was the second to wrap the left latissimus dorsi muscle around the heart.[2] Other authors have participated in this effort of transmuting a dream into reality. Leriche repaired myocardial defects in dogs with free muscle grafts,[3] Beck used pedicled muscle grafts in the human to enhance myocardial vascularization,[4] and Petrovsky resected and repaired over 100 cardiac aneurysms with diaphragmatic flaps.[5] However, none of these operations comprised a muscle stimulation, and all had the limited aim of a plastic repair.

The use of the mechanical power of skeletal muscle to assist the heart was quite a different challenge. Early attempts in the 1960s by Kantrowitz, using electrically stimulated diaphragmatic flaps,[6] and by Termet, using stimulated latissimus dorsi flaps,[7] opened the way to more extensive work by Nakamura,[8] Kusaba,[9] Macoviak and Stephenson,[10] Dewar and Chiu,[11] and others. All, however, have been facing the irritating problem of muscle fatigue, and although they could obtain efficient cardiac assistance, it lasted only a few days or weeks. From the pioneering work of Salmons[12,13] and Pette[14] it was known that the fatigable fast-twitch muscular fibers of the skeletal muscle could be transformed into fatigue-resistant slow-twitch fibers by slow rate electrical stimulation.[12–14] This muscle plasticity resulting from the capacity of the gene to code various myosin isoforms is certainly one of the most remarkable discoveries of the past decades. Could it be possible to obtain the same transformation with stimulation at heart frequency rates? Would this transformation remain stable and efficient for many years? Research was initiated in our laboratory in 1982 with the aim of finding an answer to these questions. We found that fatigue resistance of the muscle at high rate contraction could be obtained after 6 weeks by progressive training of the muscle using an original protocol of progressive sequential stimulation and that long-term cardiac assistance remained effective.[15,16]

In January 1985, a 37-year-old woman in desperate condition was admitted to Hôpital Broussais with a presumptive diagnosis of evolving constrictive pericarditis. At emergency sternotomy, a large pericardial tumor was discovered but could not be removed. Further investigations showed that the tumor had invaded the posterior wall of both ventricles, the diaphragm, and the dome of the liver. At the same time, in our research laboratory, two goats were still living and well after several months of continuous high rate contractions of an electrostimulated latissimus dorsi wrapped around the heart.

ix

A desperate medical need often hastens the transfer of research from the laboratory to clinical practice.

The operation took place on January 15, 1985 and lasted 11 hours.[17] Knowing that the removal of the tumor would leave a large myocardial defect and therefore would impair ventricular contractility, the left latissimus dorsi was dissected and transferred into the left chest. Then, performing a sternolaparotomy, a 1.8-kg tumor was removed with en-bloc resection of the posterior wall of both ventricles, the central portion of the diaphragm and the left phrenic nerve with its satellite lymph nodes. The right coronary artery was ligated to control bleeding. The diaphragm was then repaired with a large Dacron patch and the ventricular defects covered with the latissimus dorsi flap. The postoperative period required inotropic support during the 6-week program of sequential stimulation. The patient was discharged from the hospital 7 weeks following the operation. She is still living and well 5 years later with no medications.

At the time of the first International Meeting on Dynamic Cardiomyoplasty in Paris on June 1989, over 50 operations had been carried out worldwide including the 20 performed at Hôpital Broussais. It might seem presumptuous to publish a book on a nascent technique, the efficiency and the future of which has been seriously questioned by some of the most qualified experts in the field.[18,19] However, based on the preliminary results reported in this book and with further improvements to be expected, I believe that this operation will gain a significant place in surgery as an alternative to cardiac transplantation. At the very least, it is worthwhile discussing it and providing the necessary information for those who would like to participate in its development. This is precisely the purpose of this book. It provides the state of the art from the world experts in each of the disciplines that were instrumental in the development of dynamic cardiomyoplasty. I have little doubt that the readers will find these contributions outstanding and stimulating. Indeed, a large place has been given to surgical technique and clinical experience. Controversial and difficult to understand as they may be, the first clinical results form the reference for future progress to come, in essence a challenge to the growing lack of donors for cardiac transplantation.

Alain Carpentier, M.D., Ph.D.

References

1. Jesus FR: Bul Ass Med Puerto Rico 23:380, 1931.
2. Christ JE, Spira M: Application of latissimus dorsi muscle to the heart. Ann Plast Surg 8:118, 1982.
3. Leriche R: Essai expérimental de traitement de certains infarctus du myocarde et de l'anévrysme du coeur par une greffe de muscle strié. Bull Soc Nat Chir 59:229, 1933.
4. Beck CS: The development of a new blood supply to the heart by operation. Ann Surg 102:801, 1935.
5. Petrovsky BV: Surgical treatment of cardiac aneurysms. J Cardiovasc Surg 7:87, 1966.

6. Kantrowitz A, McKinnon W: The experimental use of the diaphragm as an auxilliary myocardium. Surg Forum 9:266, 1959.
7. Termet H, Chalencon JL, Estour E, et al: Transplantation sur le myocarde d'un muscle strié excité par pace-maker. Ann Chir Thorac Cardiovasc 5:270, 1966.
8. Nakamura K, Glenn WL: Graft of diaphragm as a functioning substitute for myocardium. J Surg Res 4:435, 1964.
9. Kusaba E, Schraut W, Sawatoni S: A diaphragmatic graft for augmenting left ventricular function: a feasibility study. Trans Am Soc Artif Int Org 19:251, 1973.
10. Macoviak J, Stephenson LW, Spielman S, et al: Replacement of ventricular myocardium with diaphragmatic skeletal muscle. Acute studies. J Thorac Cardiovasc Surg 81:519, 1981.
11. Dewar ML, Drinkwater DC, Chiu RC-J: Synchronously stimulated skeletal muscle graft for myocardial repair. J Thorac Cardiovasc Surg 87:325, 1984.
12. Salmons S, Streter FA: Significances of impulse activity in the transformation of skeletal muscle type. Nature 263:30, 1976.
13. Salmons S, Henriksson J: The adaptative response of skeletal muscle to increased use. Muscle & Nerve 4:94, 1981.
14. Pette D, Muller W, Leisner E, et al: Time dependent effects on contractile properties, fibre population, myosin light chains and enzymes of energy metabolism in intermittently and continuously stimulated fast twitch muscles of the rabbit. Pfluegers Arch 364:103, 1970.
15. Carpentier A, Chachques JC, Grandjean PA: Transformation d'un muscle squelettique par stimulation séquentielle progressive en vue de son utilisation comme substitut myocardique. C R Acad Sc Paris 301:581, 1985.
16. Chachques JC, Grandjean PA, Schwartz K, et al: Effects of latissimus dorsi dynamic cardiomyoplasty on ventricular function. Circulation 78 (suppl III):III-203, 1988.
17. Carpentier A, Chachques JC: Myocardial substitution with a stimulated skeletal muscle: first successful clinical case. Lancet 8440:1267, 1985.
18. Anderson WA, Andersen JS, Acker MA, et al: Skeletal muscle grafts applied to the heart. A word of caution. Circulation 78 (suppl III):III-180, 1988.
19. Walsh G, Chiu RC-J: Skeletal muscle for cardiac repair and assist: a historical overview. In R C-J Chiu (ed): Biochemical Cardiac Assist. Cardiomyoplasty and Muscle-Powered Devices. Mount Kisco NY Futura Publishing Company, 1986, pp 1–18.

Contents

Part I
Fundamentals

Chapter 1

Cardiomyoplasty:
A Look at the Fundamentals

Stanley Salmons, Jonathan C. Jarvis

Fatigue was once thought to be an insurmountable barrier to the use of skeletal muscle in a cardiac assist role. It is now known that in the long term adequate levels of fatigue resistance can be induced in skeletal muscle as part of an adaptive response to a change in functional demands.[1] Cardiomyoplasty represents the first clinical application of this knowledge to heart surgery.[2] With the accumulation of experience in this technique we are becoming increasingly aware of the need for a better understanding of the basic principles involved. To provide more cardiac assistance and to be able to introduce it at an earlier postoperative stage we need stimulation protocols that are based on a better knowledge of the requirements for conditioning and activation. In establishing objective criteria for patient selection we need to take account of the working conditions under which the skeletal muscle graft will operate and the way in which these will be affected by different cardiac pathologies. In this chapter we consider some of these issues in the light of current knowledge, and describe a new mathematical approach that may have both explanatory and predictive value.

Background

Skeletal muscle is a better generator of contractile work than cardiac muscle in terms of both the power it can develop during a single contraction and the force it can exert per unit cross-sectional area.[3] It was therefore reasonable to entertain the hope, as a number of early investigators did, that skeletal muscle might have potential for use in a cardiac assist role.[4] The acute experiments that they conducted were unsuccessful because skeletal muscle is not normally capable of sustaining cardiac levels of work other than for very short periods. The inadequate fatigue resistance of skeletal muscle was then assumed to be an insuperable problem. This assumption has now been challenged in a major way as a result of advances in basic science that originated nearly 30 years ago.

From *Cardiomyoplasty* edited by Alain Carpentier, MD, PhD, Juan-Carlos Chachques, MD, and Pierre Grandjean, MS © 1991. Futura Publishing Inc., Mount Kisco, NY.

The cross-reinnervation experiments of Buller, Eccles, and Eccles[5] showed that the characteristics by which we distinguish fast- from slow-contracting mammalian muscles can change, even in the adult animal. Thus, in spite of its high degree of specialization, skeletal muscle resembles some other mammalian tissues in showing plasticity of behavior. The introduction of the implantable muscle stimulator[6] made it possible to test rival hypotheses as to how this influence was mediated.[7] This work established beyond question that impulse activity in the motor nerve has a profound long-term influence on the properties of a skeletal muscle. Specifically, sustained high levels of use favor the differentiation of properties at the slow, fatigue-resistant end of the spectrum, whereas prolonged periods of low activity or inactivity favor retention of, or reversion to, a native fast state. At an early stage it was recognized that the response to electrical stimulation of the motor nerve could be regarded as adaptive in character.[8] The same capacity is also revealed—albeit to a less striking extent—in response to more physiological demands, such as endurance exercise and hypergravity; oppositely directed changes take place in response to detraining and disuse.[9] A concept has therefore emerged which was not available to the early investigators but which is crucially important to the application of skeletal muscle to cardiac assistance: that, in the long term, skeletal muscles are capable of accommodating changes in their pattern of use to a remarkable extent.

Although research into the adaptive transformation of muscle focused initially on changes in contractile speed, it was the strikingly improved resistance to fatigue that led to the revival of interest in the use of skeletal muscle to rehabilitate patients in end-stage heart failure. In this chapter we will show, among other things, that some determinants of fatigue resistance are in fact closely associated with contractile speed and that the latter has other effects whose significance in the context of cardiac assistance must not be overlooked.

Fatigue Resistance

The increased resistance to fatigue that is produced by chronic stimulation arises from a combination of two factors: a decrease in the energy requirements of the muscle and an enhanced capacity for generating that energy through aerobic routes. In energetic terms, maintaining a fast contractile speed is costly. The rapid distribution of calcium between intracellular compartments of the muscle fiber is an active process that accounts for a substantial fraction of the energy needed for contraction. But in response to chronic stimulation there is a reduction in the rate and amount of calcium uptake by sarcoplasmic reticulum (SR).[7,10] This is associated with early changes in the calcium transport ATPase in the membrane of the SR[11] and in calcium-binding proteins.[12] These changes affect the specific calcium-transporting properties of the SR, but stereological studies at the ultrastructural level have shown that the actual amounts of T-system and SR membrane also undergo a dramatic decline during the first two weeks of stimulation.[13] In addition to providing energy for the rapid release and uptake of calcium, the fast muscle fiber has to support rapid cycling of the propulsive crossbridges formed between the thick and thin filaments. This process is governed by a chemical reaction cycle involving the hydrolysis of ATP at an active site within the heavy chain of myosin, the protein of the thick filaments. In response to chronic stimulation, a transition takes place from myosin heavy and light chain isoforms of the fast muscle type to those characteristic of the slow muscle type.[14,15] The consequences of these changes have now been widely observed; they can be monitored biochemically as a reduction in Ca^{2+}-activated myosin ATPase and histochemically as a transformation from alkali-stable to alkali-labile characteristics. A reduction in ATP hydrolysis means less rapid turnover of crossbridges during contraction, with a corresponding saving in the energy cost of force production.[16] Changes in the kinetics of calcium transport and in myosin isoforms are responsible for the observed reduction in isometric contractile speed.[7] One consequence of this change in speed is that the muscle is capable of sustaining a given tension with less frequent activation, permitting further economies to be made in energy expenditure. Such a muscle is thus well adapted for the maintenance of steady levels of tension, although, this is not necessarily an advantage when the muscle is to be deployed in a cardiac assist role.

In parallel with these changes in the utilization of ATP during contraction, major changes take place in the metabolic pathways responsible for the generation of ATP. These consist of a switch from anaerobic to aerobic pathways, particularly those involved in the oxidative breakdown of fats and fatty acids.[17,18] Associated with this increased dependence on oxidative phosphorylation, there are marked increased in capillary density.[19] and mitochondrial volume fraction.[13] Thus on the one hand the stimulated muscle develops an increased capacity for oxidative phosphorylation while on the other it acquires more favorable bioenergetics of contraction as a result of changes in calcium kinetics and myosin isoforms. Acker and his colleagues[20] were able to demonstrate more efficient coupling between the development and maintenance of tension and the consumption of oxygen in such muscles by showing that chronically stimulated canine latissimus dorsi muscles consumed less oxygen per gram of tissue than control muscles for a given amount of internal work performed.

There is growing evidence that these adaptations, referred to collectively as "conditioning," are the result of regulatory events taking place at the level of the gene.[12,21,22] Together they enable ATP production to match even extreme increases in ATP utilization. This was well illustrated by a study in which ^{31}P-nuclear magnetic resonance (NMR) spectroscopy was used to monitor steady state high-energy phosphate metabolism in muscles contracting in vivo. When latissimus dorsi muscles of the dog were subjected to a series of fatigue tests of escalating severity, control muscles showed the decline in phosphocreatine and accumulation of ADP and inorganic phosphate that are the usual hallmarks of muscle fatigue. The conditions contralateral muscles showed only minimal changes.[23]

Isometric fatigue tests of this type have led to important and encouraging results, but they say little about the capacity of the muscle for performing external work at a sustained level. Using an implantable mock circulation

Acker et al.[24] provided the first real experimental evidence that skeletal muscle, configured in this case as a skeletal muscle ventricle, or SMV, could perform sustained external work at the required level. After a week of continuous pumping, SMVs in those experiments were still generating stroke work at a level intermediate between that of the canine right and left ventricles.

Cardiomyoplasty

Even while the SMV experiments were in progress, a human latissimus dorsi muscle, paced synchronously with the heart, was substituting for cardiac wall lost in the resection of a large tumor.[2] 52 operations of this type, termed cardiomyoplasty by Carpentier,[25] have now been carried out in a number of centers around the world. The great interest that this procedure has created among cardiothoracic surgeons is now accompanied by a desire for a better understanding of the fundamental science on which the technique is based.

There are two sound clinical reasons for seeking such an understanding. First, there are a number of aspects of the current methodology that have yet to be fully optimized. Second, while there are certain clear contraindications for the procedure, the clinical predictors of *success* are less easy to establish. In determining criteria for the selection of those candidates most likely to benefit from the operation it would be very helpful if there was a better understanding of the mechanical and physiological conditions under which the skeletal muscle grafts are required to operate.

While these statements would be equally true of other approaches to the use of skeletal muscle in cardiac assistance they are particularly significant in the context of cardiomyoplasty. Although the surgeon has some choice over the direction in which the fibers of the skeletal muscle graft are oriented during wrapping, the size of the heart and the thickness of the graft are not within his/her control. The load presented to the skeletal muscle graft is therefore largely predetermined, and the implications for the degree of cardiac assistance that will be available to a particular patient need to be understood.

Patterns of Stimulation for Conditioning and Activation

It may seem intuitively reasonable to adopt a gradually escalating pattern of stimulation in order to condition the muscle, progressing from single impulses to low-frequency and high-frequency bursts, and from assistance every few cardiac cycles to assistance on every cycle: the Paris group introduced just such a regime and it has been widely adopted. In the light of experience, however, it may be that this approach was commendably but needlessly conservative and that other patterns might permit useful assistance that can be introduced at an earlier stage. From a purely scientific point of view, patterns of this complexity introduce so many variables that it becomes difficult to compare other patterns or to evolve systematically towards more effective regimes. It would therefore be useful to begin to accumulate experience with simpler programs.

The requirements are not especially critical: adaptive transformation of muscle type has been shown to occur in response to a variety of stimulation patterns from continuous low-frequency trains to intermittent high-frequency bursts. For innervated muscles most reports would suggest that the end-result is similar when the patterns used deliver high aggregate numbers of impulses.[26] The responses may differ in other respects, however, including: the time course with which fatigue-resistant properties are acquired, the loss of bulk and force-generating capacity with which the process is associated[9] and the amount of damage that may be induced during the early stages of stimulation.[27] These aspects require further study.

Early introduction of assist also depends on identifying effective patterns of activation that minimize fatigue and are well tolerated by the patient. In this context, techniques that produce selective stimulation of different parts of the grafted muscle merit further study. There is currently no reason to suppose that stimulation patterns that are optimal for activation will also be optimal for conditioning, so there could well be a case for using two quite distinct patterns for these purposes: an accelerated conditioning pattern during an initial phase, and a suitable activation pattern in a subsequent phase during which conditioning would be completed.

If we had a detailed knowledge of the signaling processes that link excitation of the muscle membrane to the changes in gene expression that underlie conditioning, it would be comparatively easy to recommend patterns optimized specifically for this application. As yet we do not have that knowledge, and the questions remain open.

Postoperative Delay

Other constraints on the types of pattern used and the earliest stage at which they can be introduced arise from the need to provide a postoperative delay before the commencement of stimulation.[25] There are two distinct reasons for such a delay. The first is to allow time for the growth of collateral vessels, particularly in the distal portion of the latissimus dorsi graft, the blood supply of which is more seriously disrupted during dissection of the muscle from the chest wall. Normally there is a substantial increase in blood flow at the onset of stimulation. Mannion et al.[28] showed that this response was greatly reduced after ligation of the perforating arteries but was present again after 3 weeks of vascular recovery. The implication of this work is that it would be damaging to the muscle to commence stimulation before this stage had been reached. However, there is currently no general agreement as to the earliest time at which stimulation can be safely introduced. Experience may not transfer readily from one animal model to another because of known species differences in the blood supply of the latissimus dorsi muscle; even within species there may be difficulties in assembling a consistent picture because of inter-individual variation—in the pattern of venous drainage, for example. The nature of the stimulation is also a factor: patterns that minimize energy expenditure could be commenced earlier, and could themselves be utilized for their angiogenic effects. In the longer term, restoration of an adequate blood supply is crucially important; work from this laboratory shows that stimulation-induced changes in metabolism render the conditioned muscle almost totally dependent on oxidative pathways of energy generation, and the working capacity of such muscles will be limited by the rate of oxygen delivery.

The second reason for observing such a delay is specific to cardiomyoplasty, and that is to allow for development of proper adhesion between the graft and the ventricular wall. In theory, close physical contact without adhesion should be just as effective: in practice, this precaution is necessitated by the surgical requirement for maintaining a well-positioned graft.

Given that there has to be a delay of possibly 2 to 3 weeks before commencing stimulation, is there any value in beginning the conditioning process before grafting the muscle? Information bearing on this question has come from studies of the reversibility of the conditioning process. It is a corollary of the description of stimulation-induced type transformation as an adaptive phenomenon that muscle should respond to a reduction, as well as to an increase, in activity. Experimental work bears out this prediction. By 6 weeks of stimulation a fast muscle has acquired most of the properties of a slow, fatigue-resistant muscle, but if stimulation is discontinued at this stage, the muscle gradually regains its original character. The time course of this reversion is now known in some detail. It is more prolonged than that of the original transformation in terms of metabolism and capillary density, but more rapid for myosin isoform transitions; in other words the changes tend to take place in a "first-in, last-out" sequence.[29,30] It follows that some deconditioning of the muscle would take place during the delay enforced by the grafting procedure, but this would not necessarily be prohibitive in extent. In an undisturbed muscle, considerable fatigue resistance could be demonstrated even 3 weeks after cessation of stimulation.[31] However, fatigue resistance depends heavily on an adequate blood supply and would not be expected to emerge with any uniformity in a grafted muscle until all parts had been fully revascularized. It might be argued that prior conditioning would render the muscle more susceptible to ischemic damage, but we are not aware of any specific evidence that this is the case. The order in which a graft should be conditioned and raised was the subject of one study in which a diaphragm pedicle graft was stimulated continuously at 2 Hz immediately after grafting, 6 weeks after grafting, before and after grafting, and without grafting.[32] All the muscles showed good morphological preservation and advanced transformation, so that no preferred sequence emerged from this particular study. In the current state of knowledge, the best available answer to the question is that the few advantages that might be offered by prior conditioning would seem to be outweighed by the potential for adverse consequences.

Functional Role of the Skeletal Muscle Graft

The hemodynamic improvements that have been demonstrated following cardiomyoplasty are somewhat variable, and usually less than one would have expected from improvements in the general condition of the patient. This reflects uncertainties about the way in which the procedure actually works. First appearances suggest that an external wrap of skeletal muscle provides an accessory layer of ventricular wall whose contraction during systole assists in the ejection of blood. (Since the tendinous insertion of the latissimus dorsi muscle is normally reattached in the region of the rib resection, traction on the heart produced by shortening of the free portion of the graft might, in some circumstances, have an additional effect.) But the muscle may also function as a more or less passive biological reinforcement, preventing further dilatation of the heart and restoring more orderly cardiac contraction. Magovern, for example, has reported a reduction in paradoxical motion of the septum following cardiomyoplasty. Moreover, he and others have noted beneficial effects of cardiomyoplasty even though the pacemaker used to stimulate the latissimus dorsi graft was of a type that delivered only *single* impulses, and not the bursts of impulses that skeletal muscle needs for effective contraction. How, then, does stimulation contribute to the function of the graft? Clearly the skeletal muscle has to shorten actively if it is to share the workload of the patient's heart. If, on the other hand, it serves as a passive reinforcement, stimulation is still needed in order to maintain muscle bulk, preserve close apposition to the ventricular wall, and resist stretching since it is unlikely that residual endogenous impulse activity alone is sufficient to fulfill these functions.

In reality, the benefits of cardiomyoplasty are likely to derive from both active shortening and passive reinforcement. It would be useful to be able to predict, even in an approximate way, the contribution that could be expected from active shortening in a given individual. In the following sections we show how this problem may be approached.

Theoretical Maximum Ejection Fraction for the Skeletal Muscle Graft

There is a theoretical limit to the ejection fraction that a muscle wrap can produce, and we will consider this first. For the purposes of this calculation we assume an ideal situation in which sarcomeres in all parts of the encircling muscle are able to shorten to their maximum extent. We also assume that the cavity enclosed by the muscle is axially symmetrical, although we make no other assumptions about its actual shape. It is then not difficult to show (Appendix I) that the ejection fraction is given by:

$$\frac{\text{Initial volume} - \text{Final volume}}{\text{Initial volume}} = \Delta(2 - \Delta) \qquad (1)$$

where Δ represents the fractional shortening of each sarcomere measured in a direction perpendicular to the axis of the cavity. Sarcomeres cannot shorten without limit, and in practice, the shortening does not exceed 30%, i.e., $\Delta = 0.30$. The corresponding ejection fraction, calculated from Equation 1, is 0.51. (It is interesting that this simple calculation yields a value not far short of the ejection fraction of a normal left ventricle. The heart wall must be close to optimum in its fiber architecture and contraction kinetics, but presumably includes an axial component of contraction that is not taken into account in this calculation.)

The above calculation depends on there being adequate time for the sarcomeres to shorten fully. For heart rates up to 100 bpm the skeletal muscle graft can be stimulated to contract for a period of 250 msec during each systole. The amount of shortening that can take place in that time depends on the velocity of shortening and this, in any given muscle, is a function of the load against which the muscle is required to contract. In order to progress further it is therefore necessary to determine the force-velocity curve that describes this relationship, and to examine the way in which it changes with conditioning of the muscle.

Force-Velocity Characteristics

Until recently, no systematic study had been performed on stimulation-induced changes in force-velocity characteristics. Technical difficulties are partly to blame for this gap in our knowledge. The conventional method of generating force-velocity curves is to apply a constant load and to measure the velocity with which the muscle shortens. This approach is readily applicable to small muscles and single muscle fibers but it is subject to problems of inertia and friction; these become serious when attempts are made to scale up the apparatus for use with muscles such as the rabbit tibialis anterior muscle, which can generate tetanic forces of up to 5 kg. We have designed a new apparatus that eliminates these problems by inverting the conventional strategy: the selected velocity of shortening is predetermined by means of a hydraulic circuit and the force developed by the muscle is monitored continuously over the full range of contraction. With this apparatus we have been assembling a comprehensive set of force-length, force-frequency, force-velocity, and power-velocity curves for control muscles and muscles at different stages of conditioning. The experiments included fatigue tests in which the muscles were made to perform repeated cycles of contraction, enabling us to determine their capacity for sustained work under well-defined conditions of load, range of shortening, and pattern of activation.

Figures 1 and 2 are illustrative of the results obtained. They show force-velocity and power-velocity curves for the left and right tibialis anterior muscles of a deeply anesthetized rabbit. The left muscle had been conditioned by continuous stimulation at 10 Hz for 11 weeks; the right muscle served as a contralateral control.

In Figure 1 the chronically stimulated muscle shows a reduced maximum isometric force and an unloaded shortening velocity that, in terms of muscle lengths per second, has decreased to 25% of the control value. If these differences are removed by normalization, the two force-velocity curves are still different in shape. These changes reflect the transitions that have taken place in myosin isoforms. The power-velocity curves (Fig. 2) show how these changes

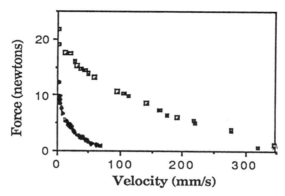

Figure 1. *Force-velocity curve of left and right tibialis anterior muscle. The left muscle (closed symbols) conditioned by continuous stimulation for 11 weeks shows a reduced maximum isometric force as compared with the nonconditioned right muscle (open symbols).*

affect the ability of the conditioned muscle to generate external work during a single contraction: the muscle shows an eight-fold reduction in power output and a five-fold reduction in the shortening velocity at which maximum power is attained. Note, however, that this maximum power is 40 W/kg, identical to the power developed by cardiac muscle during a single systolic contraction. The price paid for fatigue resistance is a substantial reduction in power output, but evidently the conditioned muscle still has the working capacity needed to perform satisfactorily in a cardiac assist role if it can be allowed to operate near to the peak of its power-velocity curve.

Working Capacity of the Skeletal Muscle Graft

These experiments show how both the loading conditions and the stage of transformation of a skeletal muscle affect the velocity at which it can

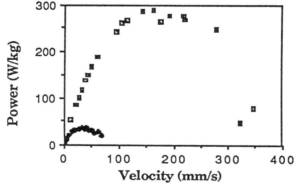

Figure 2. *Power-velocity curve shows a reduced power output of the conditioned muscle but still within the range of the power developed by cardiac muscle (40 W/kg).*

shorten, and hence its capacity for performing useful work. In order to apply the new data to muscle placed around a heart we need to know the loading conditions that the muscle will experience in this situation. This is by no means easy to predict. Laplace's Law, which is quoted widely in the cardiological literature, is helpful in understanding soap bubbles but is actually quite inappropriate to the analysis of the thick-walled cavities with which we are concerned here. It must be obvious, for example, that the inner layers of a muscular wall will be subject to greater wall tension than the outer layers, which they tend to isolate from the pressure within the cavity: Laplace's Law can make no provision for this variation in stress within the thickness of the wall. The question is, however, addressed specifically by Lamé's Equations, which are used to compute the so-called "hoop stress", σ_θ, acting tangentially within the thick walls of pressure vessels (see Appendix II). Space does not permit a full analysis here, but even a simplified analysis serves to clarify one's understanding of the issues involved.

Consider a skeletal muscle graft wrapped in a cylindrical manner around a heart of normal size. For the purposes of this calculation we will assume that the muscle acts unaided and unimpeded by the heart wall, which is therefore regarded as passive, compliant and incompressible, like a fluid. We further assume that the fibers are at ideal length and orientation throughout the graft and that length changes during contraction do not significantly alter the force and velocity that the fibers initially produce. (It is not necessary to assume that the muscle is isotropic, since we are considering only forces that are perpendicular to the long axis of the heart.) Let the inner radius of the muscle cylinder be R_i, the outer radius R_o, and the ratio of the two, $R_o/R_i = \rho$. Then the wall stress at the inner radius produced by an internal pressure P can be obtained from the cylindrical form of Lamé's Equation:

$$\sigma_\theta = P \cdot \frac{(\rho^2 + 1)}{(\rho^2 - 1)} \tag{2}$$

If $R_i = 45$ mm, then $R_o = 57$ mm, since the mean thickness reported by Chachques et al.[33] for the human latissimus dorsi muscle is 11–13 mm. If we specify a systolic pressure of 120 mm Hg, which is equivalent to 16 kN/m^2, Equation 2 gives $\sigma_\theta = 68.9$ kN/m^2. For equilibrium, this wall stress must be balanced at all times by a force generated by the muscle and therefore represents the load on the muscle. From our own work with the rabbit tibialis anterior muscle,[31] the maximum isometric force, P_o, generated per unit area is 226 kN/m^2, and the wall stress σ_θ therefore represents a fraction 0.30 of this 'specific tension.' Since the force-velocity curves were determined for the same muscle, the wall stress σ_θ also corresponds to 0.30 P_o on the force axis. At this load, the velocity is 177 mm/sec for the control muscle, and since the length of the muscle was 70.5 mm, the velocity is equivalent to 2.5 muscle lengths/sec. During a 250 msec stimulus burst the muscle should therefore shorten by a fraction $\Delta = 2.5 \times 0.25 = 0.625$. This is not possible in practice because sarcomere shortening is limited to $\Delta \leq 0.30$. We conclude that the muscle is capable of shortening to its maximum extent under these conditions. (An apparent weakness of this calculation is that it depends on force-velocity data obtained from rabbit muscle. Available figures suggest that the intrinsic speed of human muscle is not, in fact, substantially lower than represented here. Bárány[34] cites the maximum speed of shortening of human elbow flexors as 6 muscle lengths/sec. The corresponding figure was 5.2 muscle lengths/sec for the control rabbit tibialis anterior and 1.4 muscle lengths/sec for the conditioned muscle. Such species differences as do exist are likely to be less marked when comparison is made between fully conditioned muscles.) From Equation 1, ejection fraction will be 0.51, and for a left ventricular diastolic volume (LVDV) of 125 mL, the stroke volume will be 64 mL.

Consider now the conditioned muscle. The velocity corresponding to σ_θ is much lower: 23.7 mm/sec, equivalent to 0.37 muscle lengths/sec (muscle length = 64.2 mm). For a 250 msec burst the muscle shortens only by a fraction Δ = 0.092. Using Equation 1 this corresponds to an ejection fraction of 0.17. For an LVDV of 125 mL, the stroke volume will be 22 mL. In this case active assistance by the graft clearly is time-limited.

It is instructive to repeat these calculations with a larger cylinder of the type that would be needed to wrap a severely hypertrophied heart. For this purpose we set R_i = 90 mm and R_o = 102 mm (since the thickness of the latissimus graft remains at 12 mm). Entering the same systolic pressure of 16 kN/m^2 into Equation 2 now gives σ_θ = 128 kN/m^2, which is equivalent to 0.57 of the specific tension. For the control muscle, the corresponding velocity is only 70 mm/sec, or 0.99 muscle lengths/sec. In 250 msec the fractional shortening Δ = 0.25, indicating that shortening is just time-limited. The ejection fraction, from Equation 1, is 0.43. If the LVDV of this hypertrophied heart is 250 mL, the stroke volume is 108 mL.

For the conditioned muscle, however, the velocity corresponding to 0.57 of the specific tension is 7.9 mm/sec, equivalent to 0.12 muscle lengths/sec. For a 250 msec burst, Δ = 0.03, giving an ejection fraction of 0.06. With an LVDV of 250 mL, the stroke volume is 15 mL.

Interpretation ·

We should start by re-examining the assumptions and approximations that underlie these figures. First, the fiber architecture of the skeletal muscle is not optimized for the new geometry in which it finds itself, and many sarcomeres—particularly in the portion of the graft that is wrapped around the apex of the heart—will be at a suboptimal, or even nonfunctional, length. This situation will persist unless internal remodeling occurs in the long term (a possibility that deserves further study). Second, the calculation assumes that there is sufficient latissimus dorsi muscle to wrap the heart in a complete cylinder. For the heart of normal size this cylinder would have a circumference of 28 cm, which is not unreasonable in relation to a latissimus dorsi of length 33 cm. For the hypertrophied heart, the cylinder would have to have a circumference of 56 cm, which is impractical unless the muscle is used in two halves or is bridged by noncontractile tissue, such as a pericardial patch. (If a pericardial patch had to be used in wrapping the normal-sized heart, for example, and if it constituted 30% of the effective diameter, the amount of shortening that could take place after conditioning of the muscle would be reduced by 30%, and the ejection fraction would then be 0.12 instead of 0.17.) Third, it has been assumed that contraction of the graft is coupled with perfect efficiency to all parts of the left ventricle; in practice this will not be so if parts of the ventricle are not fully covered or if some of the shortening is expended in compression of the right ventricle. Fourth, substantial shortening over the declining limb of the length-tension curve must involve some reduction in force, although this may be balanced to some extent by the fall in wall tension that accompanies a reduction in diameter.

In neglecting all these factors we have *overestimated* the ability of the muscle graft to provide active assistance. However, we assumed, for this simple version of the calculation, that the heart itself was totally passive and compliant. By overlooking the contribution of the ventricular wall we have *underestimated* the capacity of the graft for providing active assistance. Until we can assess the effects of these conflicting factors quantitatively we should not take the figures too literally, but rather look at the general insights that such an approach provides.

The first clear message is that the effects of conditioning go far beyond a mere increase in the endurance of the skeletal muscle graft. The slow contractile characteristics developed by the chronically stimulated muscle severely limit the shortening that can be accommodated within a cardiac systole. Thus, a graft that functioned at a highly satisfactory level 2 weeks after operation could become much less effective after a further 2 months. This point is well illustrated by the model calculations. A point that does not emerge is that slowing also affects the rate of relaxation, creating a risk that residual tension in the muscular wrap will interfere with filling during diastole. (Commenting on this point, Professor Carpentier observed that assist was in fact more effective in some patients when the graft was activated in every other cardiac cycle rather than in every cycle.)

Is there a maximum size of heart that can be usefully assisted by cardiomyoplasty? (It was a desire to answer this question, posed by Professor Wellens (Maastricht), that prompted a mathematical analysis from which some preliminary results have been drawn for this chapter.) The calculation shows that there is a reduction in the available assistance when the heart is dilated, and although this is actually much less than the reduction that results from muscle conditioning, the two effects are additive. The difficulty of covering such a heart adequately with contractile tissue will result in a further loss of potential assistance. Thus it appears that a patient with a badly dilated heart has less to gain from cardiomyoplasty. There are, however, two other considerations. First, there is the possibility that the patient will benefit from the passive reinforcement provided by the graft. Second, if it is possible to achieve even a small ejection fraction from the graft, the stroke volume may well be appreciable because of the high LVDV of the hypertrophied ventricle. For example, an ejection fraction of 0.10 combined with an LVDV of 250 mL provides a stroke volume of 25 mL, equivalent to 2 L/min additional cardiac output at a heart rate of 80 bpm. (Professor Chiu (Montreal) has rightly emphasized that it is cardiac output, not ejection fraction, that determines whether a patient's quality of life has been improved by the procedure.)

Our scientific understanding of cardiomyoplasty has not yet advanced to the point at which it would enable us to formulate firm guidelines as to the appropriateness of this operation in individual cases. Experience with the technique continues to grow, however, and if pre- and postoperative assessment of the patients can be interpreted within the type of framework we have begun to develop here, the indications and predictors of success should become progressively more refined.

Acknowledgments: Results referred to in this chapter form part of a study supported by the British Heart Foundation. We would like to thank Mr. D.G. Moffat of the Department of Mechanical Engineering, University of Liverpool, for his advice on the application of Lamé's Equations.

APPENDIX I

For simplicity consider a cylindrical cavity of radius r and height h. The volume is given by:

$$V = \pi r^2 h$$

If the circumference shortens by a fraction Δ, it is equivalent to transforming the radius from r to $r(1 - \Delta)$. The new volume is therefore:

$$V' = \pi[r(1 - \Delta)]^2 h$$

$$\text{Ejection fraction} = \frac{V - V'}{V} = 1 - (1 - \Delta)^2$$

$$= \Delta(2 - \Delta) \tag{1}$$

This result can be generalized to any axially symmetrical cavity by generating it as the volume of a solid of revolution. If the curve $y = f(x)$ describes the wall profile, revolving it around the x-axis creates a volume:

$$V = \pi \int_a^b y^2 dx$$

in which y is the radius at any point along the axis of symmetry, x. Transforming y to $y(1 - \Delta)$ leads to:

$$V' = (1 - \Delta)^2 V$$

when Equation 1 follows as before.

APPENDIX II

When pressure P is confined to the inside of a cylindrical container of internal radius R_i and external radius R_o, Lamé's Equations[35] take the form:

$$\text{Hoop stress, } \sigma_\theta = \frac{P \cdot R_i^2}{[R_o^2 - R_i^2]} \cdot [1 + R_o^2/R^2]$$

$$\text{Radial stress, } \sigma_R = \frac{P \cdot R_i^2}{[R_o^2 - R_i^2]} \cdot [1 - R_o^2/R^2]$$

where the stresses are measured within the wall at a radius R.

References

1. Salmons S, Sréter FA: Significance of impulse activity in the transformation of skeletal muscle type. Nature 263:30, 1976.
2. Carpentier A, Chachques JC: Myocardial substitution with a stimulated skeletal muscle: first successful clinical case. Lancet 1:1267, 1985.
3. Salmons S, Jarvis JC: The working capacity of skeletal muscle transformed for use in a cardiac assist role. In RC-J Chiu, I Bourgeois (eds): Transformed Muscle for Cardiac Assist and Repair. Mount Kisco, NY, Futura Publishing Co., 1990, pp 89–104.
4. Nakamaura K, Glenn WL: Graft of diaphragm as a functioning substitute for myocardium. J Surg Res 4:435, 1964.
5. Buller AJ, Eccles JC, Eccles RM: Interactions between motoneurons and muscles in respect of the characteristic speeds of their responses. J Physiol 150:417, 1960.
6. Salmons S: An implantable muscle stimulator. J Physiol 188:13, 1967.
7. Salmons S, Vrbová G: The influence of activity on some contractile characteristics of mammalian fast and slow muscles. J Physiol 201:535, 1969.
8. Salmons S: Skeletal muscle—an adaptive machine? Brit Sci News (Spectrum) 83:2, 1971.
9. Salmons S, Henriksson J: The adaptive response of skeletal muscle to increased use. Muscle & Nerve 4:94, 1981.
10. Sréter FA, Romanul FCA, Salmons S, et al: The effect of a changed pattern of activity on some biochemical characteristics of muscle. In AT Milhorat (ed): Exploratory Concepts in Muscular Dystrophy II, Intern. Congress Series Excerpta Medica, 333:338, 1974.
11. Heilmann C, Pette D: Molecular transformations in sarcoplasmic reticulum of fast-twitch muscle by electro-stimulation. Eur J Biochem 93:437, 1979.
12. Leberer F, Seedorf U, Pette D: Neural control of gene expression in skeletal muscle. Calcium-sequestering proteins in developing and chronically stimulated rabbit skeletal muscles. Biochem J 239:295, 1986.
13. Eisenberg BR, Salmons S: Reorganisation of subcellular structure in muscle undergoing fast-to-slow type transformation: a stereological study. Cell Tiss Res 220:449, 1981.
14. Sréter FA, Gergely J, Salmons S, et al: Synthesis by fast muscle of myosin light chains characteristic of slow muscle in response to long-term stimulation. Nature 241:17, 1973.
15. Brown WE, Salmons S, Whalen RG: The sequential replacement of myosin subunit isoforms during muscle type transformation induced by long-term electrical stimulation. J Biol Chem 258:14686, 1983.
16. Crow MT, Kushmerick MJ: Chemical energetics of slow- and fast-twitch muscles of the mouse. J Gen Physiol 79:147, 1982.
17. Heilig A, Pette D: Changes induced in the enzyme activity pattern by electrical stimulation of fast-twitch muscle. In D Pette (ed), Plasticity of Muscle. Berlin, Walter de Gruyter, pp 409–420, 1980.
18. Henriksson J, Chi MM-Y, Hintz CS, et al: Chronic stimulation of mammalian muscle: changes in enzymes of six metabolic pathways. Am J Physiol 251:C614, 1986.

19. Brown MD, Cotter MA, Hudlická O, et al: The effects of different patterns of muscle activity on capillary density, mechanical properties and structure of slow and fast rabbit muscles. Pflügers Archiv 361:241, 1976.
20. Acker MA, Anderson WA, Hammond, RL, et al: Oxygen consumption of chronically stimulated skeletal muscle. J Thorac Cardiovasc Surg 94:702, 1987.
21. Williams RS, Salmons S, Newsholme EA, et al: Regulation fo nuclear and mitochondrial expression by contractile activity in skeletal muscle. J Biol Chem 261:376, 1986.
22. Brownson C, Isenberg H, Brown W, et al: Changes in skeletal muscle gene transcription induced by chronic stimulation. Muscle Nerve 11:1183, 1988.
23. Clark BJ, III, Acker MA, McCully K, et al: In vivo ^{31}P-NMR spectroscopy of chronically stimulated canine skeletal muscle. Am J Physiol 254:C258, 1988.
24. Acker MA, Hammond RL, Mannion JD, et al: An autologous biologic pump motor. J Thorac Cardiovasc Surg 92:733, 1986.
25. Carpentier A, Chachques JC, Grandjean PA, et al: Transformation d'un muscle squelettique par stimulation séquentielle progressive en vue de son utilisation comme substitut myocardique. C.R. Acad. Sc. Paris 301:581, 1985.
26. Salmons S: Re-analysis: impulse activity and fibre type transformation: a reply. Muscle Nerve 10:839, 1987.
27. Maier A, Gorza K, Schiaffino S, et al: A combined histochemical and immunohistochemical study on the dynamics of fast-to-slow fiber transformation in chronically stimulated rabbit muscle. Cell Tiss Res 254:59, 1988.
28. Mannion JD, Velchik M, Alavi A, et al: Blood flow in conditioned and unconditioned latissimus dorsi muscle. Proc 2nd Vienna International Workshop on Functional Electrostimulation, 1985, p 28.
29. Eisenberg BR, Brown JMC, Salmons S: Restoration of fast muscle characteristics following cessation of chronic stimulation: the ultrastructure of slow-to-fast transformation. Cell Tiss. Res. 238:221, 1984.
30. Brown WE, Salmons S, Whalen RG: Mechanisms underlying the asynchronous replacement of myosin light chain isoforms during stimulation-induced fibre-type transformation of skeletal muscle. FEBS Lett 192:235, 1985.
31. Brown JMC, Henriksson J, Salmons S: Restoration of fast muscle characteristics following cessation of chronic stimulation: physiological, histochemical and metabolic changes during slow-to-fast transformation. Proc R Soc B 235:321, 1989.
32. Bitto T, Mannion JD, Hammond R, et al: Preparation of fatigue-resistant diaphragmatic muscle grafts for myocardial replacement. In Y Nose, C Kjellstrand, P Ivanovich (eds): Progress in Artificial Organs, Cleveland, ISAO Press, 1986, pp 441–446.
33. Chachques JC, Grandjean PA, Carpentier A: Dynamic cardiomyoplasty: experimental cardiac wall replacement with a stimulated skeletal muscle. In RC-J Chiu (ed): Biomechanical Cardiac Assist. Mount Kisco, NY, Futura Publishing Co, 1986, pp 59–84.
34. Bárány M: ATPase activity of myosin correlated with speed of muscle shortening. J Gen Physiol 50:197, 1967.
35. Hearn EJ: Mechanics of Materials, Vol. 1, Oxford, Pergamon Press, Ltd., 1985.

Chapter 2

Changes in Phenotype Expression of Stimulated Skeletal Muscle

Dirk Pette

Since Salmons and Vrbová[1] first reported that chronic low-frequency stimulation exerts a slowing effect on rabbit fast-twitch muscle, numerous studies have addressed the question as to the molecular basis of this fast-to-slow conversion. It has now become clear that this phenomenon relates to a fundamental phenotype conversion of the stimulated muscle. Due to the variable expression of most of its proteins as various isoforms, adult skeletal muscle is capable of changing its phenotype in response to exogenous stimuli, e.g., changes in neuromuscular activity or specific hormonal signals.[2] Modifications in phenotype expression correspond to qualitative and quantitative changes in gene expression and are reflected at both the mRNA and protein levels. Studies at the mRNA level suggest that the majority of changes relate to altered transcription.[3-13] Although the fast-to-slow conversion of stimulated fast-twitch muscle primarily results from a transformation of existing fibers, it may also involve degeneration-regeneration processes with a replacement of deteriorated fibers by newly formed, satellite cell-derived myotubes.[14-16]

Chronic Stimulation Affects All Functional Elements of the Muscle Fiber

Although pronounced species-specific differences exist,[12,17,18] chronic stimulation of a fast-twitch muscle with a stimulus pattern resembling that normally delivered to a slow-twitch muscle, elicits a set of timely ordered fast-to-slow transitions that involve all functional elements of the muscle fiber. As a result, a muscle is created that, in comparison to its native phenotype, displays remarkable structural, functional, and molecular changes. Above all, the transformed muscle is characterized by slower contraction and relaxation velocities and a greatly improved resistance to fatigue. Studies at mRNA and protein levels indicate that the altered contractile properties result from changes in the Ca^{2+}-regulatory system and multiple isoform transitions of both the regulatory and contractile proteins of the myofibrillar apparatus.

From *Cardiomyoplasty* edited by Alain Carpentier, MD, PhD, Juan-Carlos Chachques, MD, and Pierre Grandjean, MS © 1991. Futura Publishing Inc., Mount Kisco, NY.

An approximate 50% decrease in the maximum rate and capacity of the Ca^{2+}-uptake by the sarcoplasmic reticulum (SR) is due to a reduced specific catalytic activity of the Ca^{2+}-ATPase of the SR soon after the onset of stimulation.[19] The decrease in Ca^{2+}-sequestration by the SR is further enhanced by a drastic reduction in parvalbumin,[5,20] the major cytosolic Ca^{2+}-binding protein of fast-twitch muscle in small mammals.[21] Ultimately, an isozyme switch with a progressive exchange of the fast SR Ca^{2+}-ATPase by its slow/cardiac isoform occurs in long-term stimulated (>35days) rabbit muscle.[22] At the same time, the expression of phospholamban, a regulatory protein of the Ca^{2+}-ATPase in heart and slow-twitch muscle, is induced in chronically stimulated fast-twitch muscle.[22]

Changes at the level of the thick and thin filaments of the myofibril are reflected by fast-to-slow transitions in the isoform patterns of myosin light and heavy chains,[3,4,9,11–13,23–27] and the three troponin subunits.[28–30] Alterations in the expression of the myosin heavy and light chains follow specific time courses.[11–13, 25–27] They precede the changes in the troponin subunit isoforms, which also follow specific time courses.[29,30] Together with data from protein analyses of single fibers,[27] these results suggest the coexistence of a large variety of isomyosins and troponin isoforms in the transforming fiber population. This is in agreement with a pronounced increase in type IC/IIC fibers (Fig. 1).[16,27]

The enhanced capacity for sustained performance relates to (1) improvements in fuel supply, and (2) quantitative and qualitative changes in enzyme activity and isozyme patterns of energy metabolism. Taken together, these metabolic transformations meet the increased ATP demand for sustained contractile activity. Thus, chronically stimulated muscle acquires properties that make it a suitable tissue for cardiac assist or cardiac repair.

Stimulation-Induced Alterations in Fuel Supply

As judged from its enzyme activity profile, rabbit fast-twitch muscle displays a glycolytically oriented metabolic phenotype. Its phasic contractile activity appears to be primarily based upon glycogen breakdown. The rapid depletion of its glycogen stores after the onset of stimulation[15] indicates that in its nonadapted state, it is metabolically unprepared to meet the energy demands for persistently increased contractile activity. The imbalance in energy supply most likely is an important factor in the deterioration of a large fraction of the fast-twitch glycolytic fibers during the first days after the onset of stimulation.[14–16] It is conceivable that fiber degeneration due to this type of metabolic imbalance is encountered less with chronic stimulation in species with higher basal aerobic-oxidative potentials than the rabbit, e.g., fast-twitch muscle of the rat.

The increased demand for fuel and oxygen supply is met by a pronounced increase in the size of the capillary bed together with an elevated maximal blood flow a few days after the onset of stimulation.[31–33] Further adaptive responses serving the augmented exchange of fuels and metabolic products

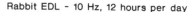

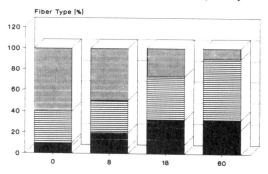

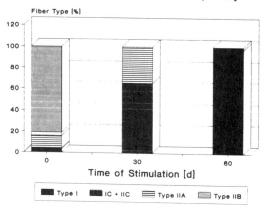

Figure 1. *Effects of two different stimulation protocols (10 Hz, 12 h/d and 10 Hz, 24 h/ d) on fiber type distribution in rabbit fast-twitch muscles. Values are from Maier et al.[16] and Staron et al.[27] EDL = extensor digitorum longus; TA = tibialis anterior.*

result in an expansion of the extracellular space[34] together with pronounced increases in extracellular albumin content.[35]

Severalfold increases in the content of free glucose in rabbit fast-twitch muscle within the first hours after the onset of stimulation suggest an enhanced glucose uptake (H.J. Green, D. Pette, unpublished results). However, as indicated by steep increases in hexokinase activity, glucose utilization appears to be limited under these conditions by the low cellular activity of this enzyme in nonadapted muscle.[36,37] Hexokinase activity is elevated 12-fold in 7-day stimulated rat muscle. This increase is confined to hexokinase II and results from enhanced synthesis. A 30-fold increase in the synthesis rate of hexokinase II was determined by in vivo labeling studies of low-frequency stimulated rat muscle.[37]

Three to fourfold increases in the content of intracellular fatty acid binding protein (FABP) occur in rat fast-twitch muscle during the first three weeks of low-frequency stimulation.[38] In combination with the elevated albumin content of the extrafibrillar interstitium,[35] this increase leads to an augmented capacity for fatty acid transport. In addition, it points to a metabolic change-over to increased fatty acid utilization. Indeed, chronic low-frequency stimulation induces pronounced increases in the activities of enzymes involved in fatty acid activation and oxidation.[18,36,38–40] According to a detailed study on rabbit muscle, this increase comprises the complete set of enzymes involved in the β-oxidative pathway, as well as carnitine palmitoyl-CoA transferase (H. Reichmann & D. Pette, unpublished results).

Stimulation-Induced Decreases in Aerobic-Oxidative Capacity

Increases in myoglobin content and in enzyme activities of aerobic substrate oxidation (the citric acid cycle, amino acid and fatty acid oxidation, respiratory chain), as well as decreases in enzyme activities of anaerobic glycogen and glucose metabolism were the first biochemical events noticed in chronically stimulated rabbit muscle.[36] A dominant role of oxidative phosphorylation for ATP supply in long-term stimulated muscle is also suggested by pronounced increments in mitochondrial content (Fig. 2). However, chronic stimulation does not only increase mitochondria by number and size[39,41,42], it alters their enzymatic composition as well.[18,40] These qualitative changes relate mainly to enzymes involved in metabolic interactions between the extra- and intramitochondrial compartments. One example of this is the severalfold increase in mitochondrial creatine kinase[43] that is interpreted to enhance the creatinephosphate-mediated export of ATP into the cytosol. Another example concerns the glycerolphosphate cycle, i.e., the decrease in the activity of mitochondrial glycerolphosphate dehydrogenase concomitant with the reduced glycolytic enzyme activities in the cytosol.[36,39] Finally, qualitative changes in

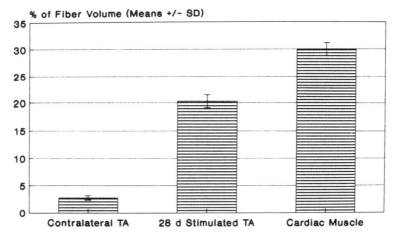

Figure 2. *Increase in mitochondrial volume density after 28 days of low-frequency stimulation (10 Hz, 12 h/d) in rabbit tibialis anterior as compared to the normal, unstimulated muscle and cardiac muscle. Values are from Reichmann et al.*[39]

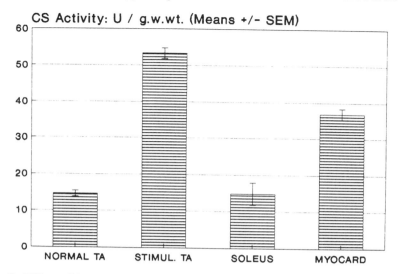

Figure 3. *Effect of long-term (>50 d) low-frequency stimulation (10 Hz, 12 h/d) on citrate synthase activity in rabbit tibialis anterior (TA) muscle. The values for normal fast-twitch TA, slow-twitch soleus, and cardiac muscle are given for comparison. Data are from Hood and Pette.[44]*

mitochondrial composition relate to pronounced increases in enzyme activities of ketone body metabolism.[18,39,40] On the whole, these changes signify an increased aerobic-oxidative capacity of the conditioned muscle. Depending on the species, long-term stimulated muscle may even attain selective properties that make it metabolically closer to cardiac muscle than to slow-twitch muscle (Fig. 3).[44]

Resistance to Fatigue

Since it was first recognized that chronic low-frequency stimulation increases resistance to fatigue,[45] this effect has often, but not exclusively, been related to the elevated aerobic-oxidative potential. Results from a recent study on rats and rabbits clearly indicate that these two parameters are not correlated throughout the entire range of adaptive responses.[46] This study compared increases in resistance to fatigue with increases in citrate synthase activity, a reference enzyme of aerobic substrate oxidation. The two parameters increased in parallel in both species during the first two weeks of low-frequency stimulation, and resistance to fatigue had reached its maximum. However, citrate synthase activity continued to increase. Obviously, a muscle must not be stimulated to the point of maximally elevated enzyme activities of aerobic-oxidative metabolism to attain maximum resistance to fatigue. Furthermore, it is evident that the fatigue characteristics of the conditioned muscle are not solely dictated by its aerobic-oxidative potential, but that additional factors, e.g., fuel supply and extra-intracellular exchange of fuels and metabolic products, may be important.

Dose-Response Relationships

With the use of different stimulation protocols, e.g., 8, 12, or 24 hours of daily stimulation, dose-response relationships have emerged with regard to metabolic changes[24] or fast-to-slow transitions. For example, 50-day intermittently (10 Hz, 8 h/d) stimulated rabbit fast-twitch muscle displays a pronounced IIB to IIA fiber type conversion without noticeable increase in the percentage of type I fibers.[47] However, increasing the daily period of stimulation leads to more extensive transformations with progressive increases in type I fibers.[16] An almost complete type II to type I conversion is observed after 60 days of continuous (24 h/d) stimulation (Fig. 1).[27]

Species-Specific Responses

Most of the previously discussed effects of chronic low-frequency stimulation apply to the rabbit. However, identical stimulus patterns may evoke variable responses in different species. Such differences could suggest the existence of various adaptive ranges due to different intrinsic properties of homologous muscles in various mammals.[18] Alternately, they could indicate species-specific thresholds, such that stimulus patterns found to be appropriate to induce changes in one species are inappropriate in other species. Therefore, species differences have to be taken into account, and further studies are necessary to elaborate optimal stimulation protocols for different species.

Species-related differences in response to chronic low-frequency stimulation were convincingly documented by studies of changes in enzyme activities of energy metabolism.[18,48] These studies included tibialis anterior muscles of four small mammals (mouse, rat, guinea pig, and rabbit) subjected to 10-Hz stimulation during identical time periods. Pronounced differences existed between the extent of decreases in glycolytic enzyme activities and increases in enzyme activities of aerobic substrate oxidation (Fig. 4). A major result was that increases in enzyme activities of aerobic substrate oxidation were inversely related to the basal levels of the aerobic-oxidative potential in the unstimulated muscles[18] Thus, increases in enzyme activities of aerobic-oxidative metabolism were highest in the rabbit and lowest in the mouse (Fig. 4). Studies performed on larger mammals, e.g., dog[49] and sheep (U. Carraro, D. Pette, unpublished results), indicate that chronic stimulation produces much smaller increments in mitochondrial enzyme activities in these animals than in the rabbit. The pronounced increases of these enzyme activities in the rabbit probably reflect the fact that due to its sedentary life-style, its skeletal muscles represent a maximally detrained state and, therefore, respond more strongly than the muscles of animals with higher spontaneous locomotor activities.

Another example of species-specific responses to low-frequency stimula-

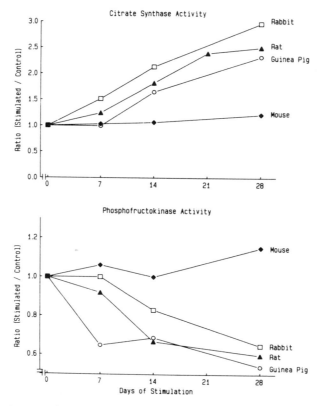

Figure 4. *Species-specific effects of low-frequency stimulation (10 Hz, 10h/d) on the activity levels of phosphofructokinase and citrate synthase in tibialis anterior muscles of four small mammals. Changes in enzyme activities were referred to the basal levels in the unstimulated muscles and are given as ratios. Values are taken from Simoneau and Pette.*[18]

tion relates to alterations in the expression of myosin heavy chain (MHC) isoforms. Whereas long-term stimulation of rabbit fast-twitch muscle ultimately leads to a complete exchange of the fast MHC with the slow MHC isoform,[25,27] an incomplete fast-to-slow conversion is found in chronically stimulated rat muscle.[11,50] Stimulation up to 7 weeks does not appreciably increase the relative concentration of the slow MHC, but evokes a rearrangement of the three fast MHC isoforms expressed in the rat. This rearrangement consists of a decrease in MHCIIb and increases in MHCIIa and MHCIId, the latter representing an isoform intermediate between MHCIIb and MHCIIa.[50,51] Complete fast-to-slow transitions in myosin expression have been reported for long-term stimulated muscles of goat,[52] dog,[49] and sheep.[53]

Time Course and Reversibility of Changes

Chronic low-frequency stimulation induces reversible changes in phenotype expression.[54,55] As judged from physiological and biochemical studies, stimulation-induced changes and their reversion after cessation of stimulation follow specific time courses. Some changes are detectable a few hours after the onset of stimulation, e.g., the reduced Ca^{2+}-uptake by the SR (L. Dux, D. Pette, unpublished results). Other changes manifest themselves after longer stimulation periods, e.g., transitions of myofibrillar protein isoforms. Emerging evidence indicates that the onset of these changes may occur earlier than previously thought and may have escaped detection in previous studies. Pronounced alterations in MHC expression are detectable at the mRNA level in rat muscle as soon as two days after the onset of stimulation.[11] These changes consist of progressive increases in MHCIIa mRNA content at the expense of MHCIIb mRNA, the latter decreasing after 7 days to barely detectable levels. Cessation of stimulation leads to a progressive reappearance of MHCIIb mRNA concomitant with a decrease in MHCIIa mRNA. The reappearance of MHCIIb mRNA is detectable as soon as 21 hours after cessation of stimulation (ref. 11, and unpublished results).

Another example illustrating the rapid time course of a stimulation-induced change and its reversion concerns hexokinase II. As discussed previously, a 12-fold rise in total hexokinase activity in 7-day stimulated rat muscle results from a drastic increase in the synthesis rate of the enzyme.[37] However, the synthesis rate is reduced to normal values within approximately 15 hours after cessation of stimulation (unpublished results). The elevated level of hexokinase II is still unaltered by this time, probably because its degradation is slow and does not involve specific mechanisms.

Conclusions

Increased neuromuscular activity as imposed by low-frequency stimulation induces profound changes in phenotype expression in mammalian fast-twitch muscle and leads to conversion to a slow-contracting muscle with an enhanced resistance to fatigue. The conversion affects all functional elements of the muscle fiber studied to date. The changes follow specific time courses, reveal dose-response relationships, and are reversible after cessation of stimulation. Studies of alterations in myosin heavy chain expression at the mRNA level and measurements of relative synthesis rates of hexokinase II indicate that stimulation-induced changes may follow much faster time courses than previously thought. Finally, species-specific responses suggest the existence of variable adaptive ranges, but could also indicate that different stimulus patterns must be used to evoke maximal responses in different species.

References

1. Salmons S, Vrbová G: The influence of activity on some contractile characteristics of mammalian fast and slow muscles. J Physiol (Lond) 201:535, 1969.
2. Pette D, Vrbová G: Neural control of phenotypic expression in mammalian muscle fibers. Muscle Nerve 8:676, 1985.
3. Heilig A, Pette D: Changes in transcriptional activity of chronically stimulated fast twitch muscle. FEBS Lett 151:211, 1983.

4. Pluskal MG, Sréter FA: Correlation between protein phenotype and gene expression in adult rabbit fast twitch muscles undergoing a fast to slow fiber transformation in response to electrical stimulation in vivo. Biochem Biophys Res Commun 113:325, 1983.

5. Leberer E, Seedorf U, Pette D: Neural control of gene expression in skeletal muscle. Ca-sequestering proteins in developing and chronically stimulated rabbit skeletal muscles. Biochem J 239:295, 1986.

6. Seedorf U, Leberer E, Kirschbaum BJ, et al: Neural control of gene expression in skeletal muscle. Effects of chronic stimulation on lactate dehydrogenase isoenzymes and citrate synthase. Biochem J 239:115, 1986.

7. Williams RS, Salmons S, Newsholme EA, et al: Regulation of nuclear and mitochondrial gene expression by contractile activity in skeletal muscle. J Biol Chem 261:376, 1986.

8. Williams SR, Garcia-Moll M, Mellor J, et al: Adaptation of skeletal muscle to increased contractile activity. Expression of nuclear genes encoding mitochondrial proteins. J Biol Chem 262:2764, 1987.

9. Brownson C, Isenberg H, Brown W, et al: Changes in skeletal muscle gene transcription induced by chronic stimulation. Muscle Nerve 11:1183, 1988.

10. Hood DA, Zak R, Pette D: Chronic stimulation of rat skeletal muscle induces co-ordinate increases in mitochondrial and nuclear mRNAs of cytochrome c oxidase subunits. Eur J Biochem 179:275, 1989.

11. Kirschbaum BJ, Simoneau J-A, Pette D: Dynamics of myosin expression during the induced transformation of adult rat fast-twitch muscle. Cellular and molecular biology of muscle development. In F Stockdale, L Kedes (eds): UCLA Symposia on Molecular and Cellular Biology, New Series, Vol 93. New York, Alan R Liss, Inc, 1989, pp 461–469, 1989.

12. Kirschbaum BJ, Heilig A, Härtner K-T, Pette D: Electrostimulation-induced fast-to-slow transitions of myosin light and heavy chains in rabbit fast-twitch muscle at the mRNA level. FEBS Lett 243:123, 1989.

13. Kirschbaum BJ, Simoneau J-A, Bär A, et al: Chronic stimulation-induced changes of myosin light chains at the mRNA and protein levels in rat fast-twitch muscle. Eur J Biochem 179:23, 1989.

14. Maier A, Gambke B, Pette D: Degeneration-regeneration as a mechanism contributing to the fast to slow conversion of chronically stimulated fast-twitch rabbit muscle. Cell Tissue Res 244:635, 1986.

15. Maier A, Pette D: The time course of glycogen depletion in single fibers of chronically stimulated rabbit fast-twitch muscle. Pflügers Arch 408:338, 1987.

16. Maier A, Gorza L, Schiaffino S, et al: A combined histochemical and immunohistochemical study on the dynamics of fast to slow fiber transformation in chronically stimulated rabbit muscle. Cell Tissue Res 254:59, 1988.

17. Kwong WH, Vrbová G: Effects of low-frequency electrical stimulation on fast and slow muscles of the rat. Pflügers Arch 391:200, 1981.

18. Simoneau J-A, Pette D: Species-specific effects of chronic nerve stimulation upon tibialis anterior muscle in mouse, rat, guinea pig, and rabbit. Pflügers Arch. 412:86, 1988.

19. Leberer E, Härtner K-T, Pette D: Reversible inhibition of sarcoplasmic reticulum Ca-ATPase by altered neuromuscular activity in rabbit fast-twitch muscle. Eur J Biochem 162:555, 1987.

20. Klug GA, Leberer E, Leisner E, et al: Relationship between parvalbumin content and the speed of relaxation in chronically stimulated rabbit fast-twitch muscle. Pflügers Arch 411:126, 1988.

21. Heizmann CW, Berchtold MW, Rowlerson AM: Correlation of parvalbumin concentration with relaxation speed in mammalian muscles. Proc Natl Acad Sci USA 79:7243, 1982.

22. Leberer E, Härtner K-T, Brandl CJ, et al: Slow/cardiac sarcoplasmic reticulum Ca-ATPase and phospholamban mRNAs are expressed in chronically stimulated rabbit fast-twitch muscle. Eur J Biochem 185:51, 1989.

23. Sréter FA, Gergely J, Salmons S, et al: Synthesis by fast muscle of myosin light chains characteristic of slow muscle in response to long-term stimulation. Nature (London) 241:17, 1973.
24. Pette D, Müller W, Leisner E, et al: Time dependent effects on contractile properties, fibre population, myosin light chains and enzymes of energy metabolism in intermittently and continuously stimulated fast twitch muscle of the rabbit. Pflügers Arch 364:103, 1976.
25. Brown WE, Salmons S, Whalen RG: The sequential replacement of myosin subunit isoforms during muscle type transformation induced by long term electrical stimulation. J Biol Chem 258:14686, 1983.
26. Seedorf K, Seedorf U, Pette D: Coordinate expression of alkali and DTNB myosin light chains during transformation of rabbit fast muscle by chronic stimulation. FEBS Lett 158:321, 1983.
27. Staron RS, Gohlsch B, Pette D: Myosin polymorphism in single fibers of chronically stimulated rabbit fast-twitch muscle. Pflügers Arch 408:444, 1987.
28. Schachat FH, Williams RS, Schnurr CA: Coordinate changes in fast thin filament and Z-line protein expression in the early response to chronic stimulation. J Biol Chem 263:13975, 1988.
29. Härtner K-T, Kirschbaum BJ, Pette D: The multiplicity of troponin T isoforms. Normal rabbit muscles and effects of chronic stimulation. Eur J Biochem 179:31, 1989.
30. Härtner K-T, Pette D: Effects of chronic low-frequency stimulation on troponin I and troponin C isoforms in rabbit fast-twitch muscle. Eur J Biochem (submitted).
31. Hudlická O, Dodd L, Renkin EM, et al: Early changes in fiber profile and capillary density in long-term stimulated muscles. Am J Physiol 243:H528, 1982.
32. Hudlická O, Cotter MA, Cooper J: The effect of long- term electrical stimulation on capillary supply and metabolism in fast skeletal muscle. In WA Nix, G Vrbová (eds): Electrical Stimulation and Neuromuscular Disorders. Berlin, Heidelberg, New York, Springer, 1986, pp 21–32A 1986.
33. Hudlická O, Hoppeler H, Uhlmann E: Relationship between the size of the capillary bed and oxidative capacity in various cat skeletal muscles. Pflügers Arch 410:369, 1987.
34. Henriksson J, Salmons S, Chi M M-Y, et al: Chronic stimulation of mammalian muscle: changes in metabolite concentrations in individual fibers. Am J Physiol 255:C543, 1988.
35. Heilig A, Pette D: Albumin in rabbit skeletal muscle. Origin, distribution and regulation by contractile activity. Eur J Biochem 171:503, 1988.
36. Pette D, Smith ME, Staudte HW, et al: Effects of long-term electrical stimulation on some contractile and metabolic characteristics of fast rabbit muscles. Pflügers Arch 338:257, 1973.
37. Weber FE, Pette D: Contractile activity enhances the synthesis of hexokinase II in rat skeletal muscle. FEBS Lett 238:71, 1988.
38. Kaufmann M, Simoneau J-A, Veerkamp JH, et al: Electrostimulation-induced increases in fatty acid- binding protein and myoglobin in rat fast-twitch muscle and comparison with tissue levels in heart. FEBS Lett 245:181, 1989.
39. Reichmann H, Hoppeler H, Mathieu-Costello O, et al: Biochemical and ultrastructural changes of skeletal muscle mitochondria after chronic electrical stimulation in rabbits. Pflügers Arch 404:1, 1985.
40. Henriksson J, Chi M M-Y, Hintz CS, et al: Chronic stimulation of mammalian muscle: changes in enzymes of six metabolic pathways. Am J Physiol 251:C614-C632, 1986.
41. Eisenberg BR, Salmons S: The reorganization of subcellular structure in muscle undergoing fast-to-slow type transformation. A stereological study. Cell Tissue Res 220:449, 1981.
42. Hoppeler H, Hudlická O, Uhlmann E: Relationship between mitochondria and oxygen consumption in isolated cat muscles. J Physiol (London) 385:661, 1987.

43. Schmitt T, Pette D: Increased mitochondrial creatine kinase in chronically stimulated fast-twitch rabbit muscle. FEBS Lett 188:341, 1985.
44. Hood DA, Pette D: Chronic long-term stimulation creates a unique metabolic enzyme profile in rabbit fast-twitch muscle. FEBS Lett 247:471, 1989.
45. Peckham PH, Mortimer JT, van der Meulen JP: Physiologic and metabolic changes in white muscle of cat following induced exercise. Brain Res 50:424, 1973.
46. Simoneau J-A, Kaufmann M, Pette D: Relations between chronic stimulation-induced changes in aerobic-oxidative metabolism and resistance to fatigue of rat and rabbit fast-twitch muscles. Pfluegers Arch 414:629, 1989.
47. Mabuchi K, Szvetko D, Pinter K, et al: Type IIB to IIA fiber transformation in intermittently stimulated rabbit muscles. Am J Physiol 242:C373, 1982.
48. Simoneau J-A, Pette D: Species-specific responses of muscle lactate dehydrogenase isozymes to increased contractile activity. Pflügers Arch 413:679, 1989.
49. Acker MA, Mannion JD, Brown WE, et al: Canine diaphragm muscle after 1 yr of continuous electrical stimulation: its potential as a myocardial substitute. J Appl Physiol 62:1264, 1987.
50. Termin A, Staron RS, Pette D: Changes in myosin heavy chain isoforms during chronic low-frequency stimulation of rat fast hind limb muscles—A single fiber study. Eur J Biochem 186:749, 1989.
51. Schiaffino S, Ausoni S, Gorza L, et al: Myosin heavy chain isoforms and velocity of shortening of type 2 skeletal muscle fibres. Acta Physiol Scand 134:575, 1988.
52. Carpentier A, Chachques JC, Grandjean P: Transformation d'un muscle squelettique par stimulation sequentielle progressive en vue de son utilisation comme substitut myocardique. C.R. Acad Sc Paris 30:581, 1985.
53. Carraro U, Catani C, Dell'Antone P, et al: An experimental pumping chamber made in situ with sheep latissimus dorsi: light microscopy and isomyosins. In U Carraro (ed): Sarcomeric and Non-Sarcomeric Muscles: Basic and Applied Research Prospects for the90's. Padova, Unipress, 1988, pp 459–470.
54. Eisenberg BR, Brown JMC, Salmons S: Restoration of fast muscle characteristics following cessation of chronic stimulation. The ultrastructure of slow-to-fast transformation. Cell Tissue Res 238:221, 1984.
55. Brown JMC, Henriksson J, Salmons S: Restoration of fast muscle characteristics following cessation of chronic stimulation: physiological, histochemical and metabolic changes during slow-to-fast transformation. Proc R Soc Lond B 235:321, 1989.

Chapter 3

Isomyosins in Stimulated Skeletal Muscle

Ugo Carraro, Giorgio Arpesella

A skeletal muscle pumping chamber (SMPC) was constructed in adult sheep by freeing the left latissimus dorsi (LD) and wrapping it around a plastic bladder. After a week of healing, the SMPC was conditioned by gradually escalating the stimulation protocol, which began with a 10-Hz continuous pattern. At the end of the 3-week conditioning, the SMPC was stimulated 24 hours a day at 30 Hz with a duty cycle of 125 msec ON 1,000 msec OFF. Histochemical and biochemical analyses were performed on muscle biopsies taken at the time of the SMPC construction and 2, 14, and 16 weeks later. Histological and histochemical examination of muscle samples from SMPC revealed some muscle atrophy and dystrophy early after surgery. The muscle then became more trophic and showed an increased oxidative capacity. The increase in the proportion of fatigue-resistant type I fiber (up to 100%) compared to the 10%–20% in the control preconditioned LD samples become evident 14 weeks after operation. Accordingly, analyses of isomyosins by (1) polyacrylamide gel electrophoresis under nondissociating conditions and (2) SDS PAGE and SDS Orthogonal Peptide Mapping (SDS OPM) of myosin heavy chains, according to Carraro and Catani, showed that the fast types were eliminated, leaving only the slow type I isoform. However, the ability to sustain cardiaclike work was acquired during the second week of muscle conditioning. Our results suggest that a delay of several weeks before full strength muscle activation in cardiomyoplasty and related applications is unnecessary and probably self-defeating.

Methods

Adult sheep were used in all experiments. Under general anesthesia, a cutaneous incision was made in the subscapular dorsal region in an antero-

Supported by funds from the C. N. R. and the Ministero della Pubblica istruzione.
From *Cardiomyoplasty* edited by Alain Carpentier, MD, PhD, Juan-Carlos Chachques, MD, and Pierre Grandjean, MS © 1991. Futura Publishing Inc., Mount Kisco, NY.

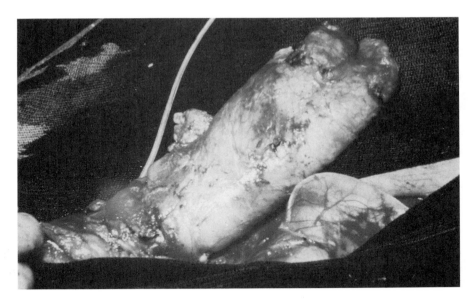

Figure 1. *Skeletal muscle pumping chamber made in situ with sheep LD.*

lateral direction toward the posterior axillary line. Subcutaneous muscles were incised resulting in the superior plane of LD and the muscle being isolated on all sides except the principal pedicle (vascular and nervous components), which remained connected to the animal. The muscle was implanted with modified Sorin electrodes and an Itrel™ programmable neurostimulator (Medtronic Model 7420) essentially according to Carpentier et al. [1,2] The anode was split in two branches and placed close to the nerve entrances into the LD, and the cathode was placed distally in the muscle. The SMPC was constructed essentially according to Acker et al.[3] by wrapping the free LD muscle around and fitting it to a Dacron-covered silicone system of three closed tubes filled with a sterile solution. The central cylinder was equipped with a pressure line ending with a subcutaneous chamber for percutaneous monitoring of pressure. This pressure port permitted measurement of pressure produced by the SMPC (Fig. 1). After 8 days of healing, the sheep was gradually introduced to electrostimulation by switching the stimulator on at 10 Hz, with a pulse width of 0.22 ms, continuous mode, for 2 hours a day for the next 4 days. LD conditioning to fatigue resistance then continued following the escalating protocol described in Table 1.

Histochemical and biochemical analyses were performed on muscle biopsies taken at the time of the SMPC construction and several weeks later. Purification of myosin, one-dimensional analysis and orthogonal peptide mapping in sodium dodecyl sulfate-polyacrylamide gel electrophoresis (SDS PAGE; SDS OPM) of myosin heavy chains (MHC) from muscle fragments were as described in Carraro et al.[4-6] N-acetyl-glucosaminidase, used as a marker for

Table 1
Stimulation Protocol

Days	Hz	Mode/Time (h/day)	ON–OFF (sec)	Tetani/Min	Tetani/d
0–8	healing	–	–	–	–
8–12	10	contin./2 h	–	–	–
12–16	10	contin./24 h	–	–	–
16–20	10	cycling/24 h	0.125–4	(sub)14	(sub)20,160
20–24	30	cycling/24 h	0.125–4	14	20,160
24–28	30	cycling/24 h	0.125–2	28	40,320
28–x	30	cycling/24 h	0.125–1	53	80,640

lysosomal content of the muscle tissue, was measured as described by Dell'Antone.[7]

Results and Discussion

SMPC constructed with sheep LD has the ability to perform 60 contractions/min 24 h a day for an extended period of time. After several weeks of such activity, the LD muscle fibers at molecular level exhibit characteristics that are peculiar to the slow fatigue-resistant type.[8] There is a substantial increase in the proportion of fatigue-resistant type I fiber (up to 100%), compared to the 10%–20% in the control preconditioned LD muscle samples. Polyacrylamide gel electrophoresis under nondissociating conditions of myosin showed that the fast types were eliminated, leaving only the slow-type isoform. The analysis of stimulated LD muscle after staining for myofibrillar ATPase activities shed some light on the cellular processes of transformation of the muscle. The original fast pattern of LD muscle is unchanged after 2 weeks of electrostimulation, while after 14–16 weeks, the slow fibers prevail. However, atrophic fast fibers are always recognizable, as well as some disarrangement of the tissue. Activity of lysosomal enzymes, biochemical markers of muscle dystrophy, however, is not increased in long-term stimulated LD muscle (N-acetyl-glucosaminidase activity nmol/min/mg protein at 37°C: control LD 0.57 +/– 0.18 SD vs 0.98 +/– 0.63 SD stimulated LD muscle, not a significant difference after ANOVA variance analysis). A differential atrophy of fast fibers certainly contributes to the dramatic decrease of the fast myosin in the long-term electrostimulated muscles, but transformation of pre-existing fibers also plays a significant role. Transient atrophy of portions of the muscle mass can be the consequence of the tenotomy that cannot be completely reversed during SMPC construction. However, this cannot be accepted as an explanation of the atrophy of the fast fibers scattered among hypertrophic slow fibers, unless one is reminded that in quiescent (by denervation or tenotomy) mixed muscles the fast fibers are initially the most sensitive to disuse.

SDS PAGE and SDS OPM of myosin heavy chains confirm the transformation of the isomyosin patterns in long-term stimulated LD muscle. There is a substantial increase in the proportion of fatigue-resistant type I MHC (up to 100%), compared to the 10%–20% in the control preconditioned LD samples (Fig. 2 and Table 2).

However, during these experiments we had further evidence that a muscle becomes capable of sustaining continuous (24 h/day) tetanic/cardiaclike work during the second week of muscle conditioning. This clinically relevant observation is substantiated by a long list of published experimental results (see for review refs. 10, 11) and by our experiments on rat muscles,[5,6] which confirm that the isomyosin transformation is the product of the long-term continuously increased demand on muscle, not a prerequisite. Indeed, isomyosin shift from the fast (whatever their myosin heavy chain composition is, either 2B, 2A, or the newly discovered fast-type myosin heavy chain) to the slow type, although useful to increase muscle efficiency (lower ATP consumption per tetanus) is not required in order to use skeletal muscle as a cardiac substitute. Stephenson's[3] recognition of the relevance of experimental evidence of exercise-drive muscle plasticity to the use of skeletal muscle in cardiac assistance and the first successful clinical myocardial substitution with a stimulated skeletal muscle by Carpentier[1] started the modern era of this approach to heart failure treatment. The success of muscle training by sequential progressive stimulation counterbalances the failures due to fatigue that frustrated the pioneers of this technique. Low-frequency, continuous stimulation protocols (mimicking those used in academic experiments had been used, and the belief still exists that several weeks of training is necessary before skeletal muscle can sustain a continuous cardiaclike performance. The basis for this belief is experimental evidence that several weeks (at least 10) of continuous exercise are necessary to obtain the half-transformation of contractile proteins in a fast-fatigable muscle to the slow, fatigue-resistant type. It is questionable if structural changes at the contractile protein level are an absolute prerequisite to allow skeletal muscle to sustain cardiaclike function. Indeed, long before there are major changes in contractile proteins, the LD muscle is able to sustain 125 ms long tetanic contractions. 60/min, 24 hours a day. As shown in Table 3, this performance, which is the consequence of changes occurring early after the onset of the newly increased work demand on the muscle calcium control, oxidative capacity, and vascularization,[10,11] may be acquired during the first week of continuous exercise in a protocol of accelerated muscle conditioning.

As a consequence, it can be predicted that our observations will be confirmed by independent researchers and that early after surgery it will be possible with an escalating cycling protocol to obtain a low, but significant amount of function, which could be used for cardiac support and to drive changes of muscle characteristics. During the muscle conditioning, it will be possible to increase the frequency of the tetanic contractions every second day or even earlier and then the frequency of train impulses so that the muscle will be able to bear higher and higher amounts of work without measurable signs of

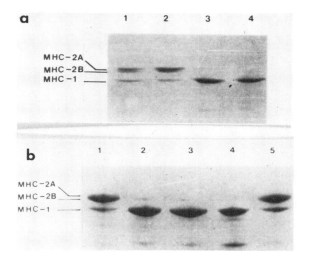
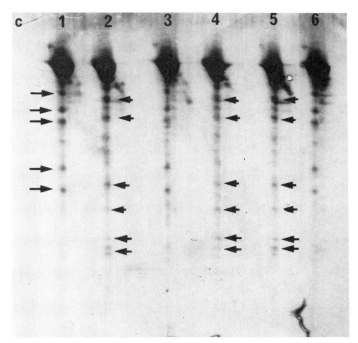

Figure 2. SDS 6% PAGE and SDS OPM of myosin heavy chains of sheep LD after completion of the pumping chamber. a. SDS 6% PAGE of MHC from sheep 2-87: (1) proximal sample, (2) laterodistal sample of LD at the time of operation; (3) proximal sample, (4) laterodistal sample of LD 17 weeks later; b. SDS 6% PAGE of MHC from sheep 1-88: (1) LD at the time of operation; (2) proximal sample, (3) laterodistal sample of LD 15 weeks later; (4) soleus; (5) peroneus. c. SDS OPM of MHC from: sheep 2-87 (1) LD at the time of operation and (2) 17 weeks later; sheep 1-88: (3) sample of LD at the time of operation and (4) 15 weeks later; (5) soleus; (6) peroneus. MHC-2A-myosin heavy chain of type IIA fiber; MHC-2B-myosin heavy chain of type IIB fiber; MHC-1-myosin heavy chain of type I fiber. Arrows pointing to the right identify peptide fragments derived from fast MHC; arrows pointing to the left indicate peptide fragments derived from slow MHC.

Table 2
Slow MHC Content of Sheep LD Muscle after
the Pumping Chamber Completion

Sheep	Electrostimulation (weeks)	MHC 1 (slow type) (%)
2-88	0	16
3-88	0	19
1-87	0	13
	2	30
1-89	0	2
	8	14
2-89	0	10
	12	51
1-88	0	23
	14	95
2-87	0	22
	16	93

Table 3
Stimulation Protocol, Accelerated Muscle Conditioning

Days	Frequency (Hz)(AP)	Mode/Time (h/day)	ON–OFF (msec)	Tetani/Min	Tetani/d
1	healing	–	–	–	–
2–3	20 2	cycling/24 h	125–10,000	6	864
4–7	20 2	" "	125–4,000	15	21,600
8–11	20 2	" "	125–1,000	60	86,400
12–15	43 5	" "	125–1,000	60	86,400
16–?	43 5	" "	125–375	120	172,800

fatigue. At the end of a 2-week conditioning, the amount of performance required to assist circulation could be obtained by adjusting the frequency and therefore the strength of tetanic contractions of the skeletal muscle. In conclusion, we believe that in the near future biologically activated circulation support devices will have an increasing role in reducing disability and death from heart diseases.

References

1. Carpentier A, Chachques JC, Grandjan PA: Transformation d'un muscle squelettique par stimulation sequentielle progressive en vue de son utilisation comme substitut myocardique. C.R. Acad Sc Paris 30:581, 1985.

2. Magovern GJ, Heckler FR, Park SB, et al: Paced skeletal muscle for dynamic cardiomyoplasty. Ann Thorac Surg 45:614, 1988.
3. Acker MA, Hammond RL, Mannion JD, et al: Skeletal muscle as the potential power source for a cardiovascular pump: assessment in vivo. Science 236:324, 1987.
4. Carraro U, Morale D, Mussini I, et al: Chronic denervation of rat hemidiaphragm: maintenance of fiber heterogeneity with associated increasing uniformity of myosin isoforms. J Cell Biol 100:161, 1985.
5. Carraro U, Catani C, Belluco S, et al: Slow-like electro-stimulation switches on slow myosin in denervated fast muscles. Exp Neurol 94:537, 1986.
6. Carraro U, Catani C, Saggin L, et al: Isomyosin changes after functional electrostimulation of denervated sheep muscle. Muscle Nerve 11:1026, 1988.
7. Dell'Antone P: Proton pump-linked $Mg2^{+}$-ATPase activity in isolated rat liver lysosomes. Arch Biochem Biophys 226:314, 1988.
8. Carraro U, Catani C, Dell'Antone P, et al: An experimental pumping chamber made with sheep latissimus dorsi: light microscopy and isomyosins. In U Carraro (ed): Sarcomeric and Nonsarcomeric Muscles: Basic and Applied Research Prospects for the 90's. Padova (Italy), Unipress Padova, 1988, pp 459–470.
9. Carraro U: The denervated muscle: a standby enginge. In E. Stagnaro (ed): Towards the Artificial Heart. Padova, Imprimitur, 1988, pp 179–188.
10. Salmons S, Henriksson J: The adaptive response of skeletal muscle to increased use. Muscle Nerve 4:94, 1981.
11. Pette D, Vrbova G: Neural control of phenotypic expression in mammalian muscle fibers. Muscle Nerve 8:676, 1985.

Chapter 4

Electrical Stimulation of Skeletal Muscles

Pierre A. Grandjean

The recent introduction of cardiomyoplasty in the arena of cardiac surgery[1] has generated a renewal of interest in electrical stimulation of skeletal muscles among cardiac surgeons and basic muscle physiologists. Numerous experimental works and some clinical applications involving functional muscle stimulation have been undertaken in recent years in other fields that will be reviewed here briefly with special emphasis on skeletal muscle physiology, skeletal muscle response to electrical stimulation, and the methods to stimulate them.

Skeletal Muscle Physiology[2]

Skeletal muscles are controlled by nerve impulses transmitted via nerve fibers. The muscle belly is made up of thousands of individual muscle fibers attached at each end to muscle tendons (Fig. 1a). When stimulated, the muscle fibers contract, and the force of contraction is transmitted to the bones through the tendons.

Each motor neuron that leaves the spinal cord usually innervates many different muscle fibers, the number depends on the type of muscle. All the muscle fibers innervated by a single motor nerve fiber are called a motor unit.

In general, small muscles (e.g., laryngeal muscles) that react rapidly and whose control is exact have few muscle fibers in each motor unit (2–5 per motor unit) and a large number of nerve fibers going to each muscle. Large muscles that do not require a very fine degree of control (e.g., gastrocnemius) may have several hundred muscle fibers in a motor unit. The average figure for skeletal muscles is about 150 fibers per motor unit.

A muscle can be composed of different motor unit sizes. Large motor units are innervated by large nerve fibers (10–20 μ) and, small motor units are innervated by small nerve fibers (3–10 μ).Nerve fiber and muscular fiber connect via the neuromuscular junction.

From *Cardiomyoplasty* edited by Alain Carpentier, MD, PhD, Juan-Carlos Chachques, MD, and Pierre Grandjean, MS © 1991. Futura Publishing Inc., Mount Kisco, NY.

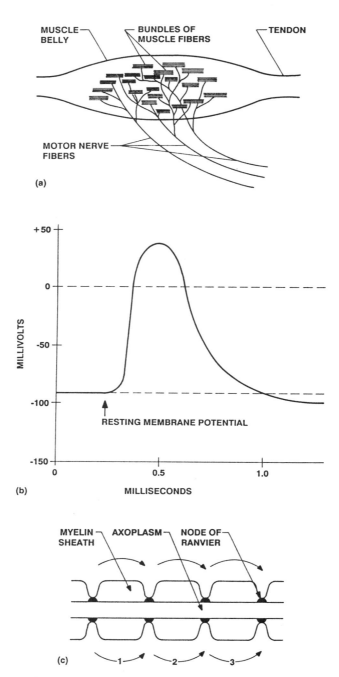

Figure 1. *Distribution of nerve fibers supplying three motor units (a), action potential transmitted along a large nerve fiber (b), and saltatory conduction process in a myelinated axon (c).*

Table 1
Nerve Fiber Types

	Fiber Types	Myelin	Fiber Diameter (μm)	Conduction Velocity (m/sec)	Spike Duration (msec)	Absolute Refractory Period (msec)	Function
Motor	A 4 Groups	With	3–20	15–120	0.4–0.5	0.4–1	Somatic motor, Motor to muscle spindle
Sensory	A 4 Groups	With	2–20	12–120	0.4–0.5	0.4–1	Pain (FAST)? proprioception Touch, Pressure and vibratory receptors
	C	Without	0.5–1	0.5–2	2	2	Temperature Pain (slow) mechanoreceptors
Motor	B	With	1–3	3–15	1.2	1.2	Preganglionic sympathetics

Nerve impulses (action potentials resulting from membrane depolarization generated by the "sodium pump" action) travel along nerve fibers (Fig.1b). Depolarization duration and refractory periods are short (0.4–2.0 ms). Propagation velocity depends on nerve fiber types (myelinated or nonmyelinated) and sizes[2] (Table 1). Conduction velocity is higher on myelinated than nonmyelinated axons due to the saltatory conduction process (Fig.1c). The distance between Ranvier nodes being proportional to axon diameter, the larger the fiber, the higher the conduction velocity. Action potential propagation is unidirectional.

When an action potential reaches the neuromuscular junction, acetylcholine is released making the muscle fiber membrane-permeable to sodium ions. The rapid influx of ions creates a local electrical current flow that, if strong enough, initiates an action potential traveling in both directions along the membrane of the muscle fiber (velocity: 5 m/sec). A muscle action potential excites the entire fiber in a very short period of time.

The action potential causes electrical current to flow toward the interior of the muscular fiber by ionic conduction through the extracellular fluid in the "T" tubules. This causes calcium ion release, which in turn causes myofibrillar contraction. Contraction of a skeletal muscle fiber following a single action potential lasts only a small fraction of a second, because after release of calcium ions into the myofibrillar fluid, the wall of the longitudinal tubules immediately begins active transport of the calcium ions back to endoplasmic fluid.

To complete this process requires only a few thousands of a millisecond in fast-acting skeletal muscles (fiber type II) such as eye muscles and only a few hundreds of a millisecond in slow-acting muscles (fiber type I) e.g., soleus.

It is during the time that calcium ions are present in sufficient quantity in the myofibrils that the muscle fiber remains contracted. Isometric contractions by muscles of different fiber compositions generated by a single action potential are shown in Figure 2a. It shows the specialization and/or adaptation

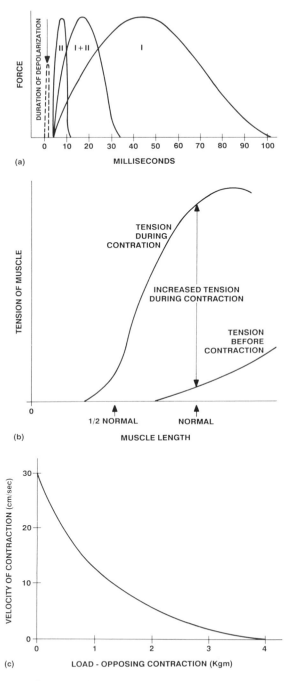

Figure 2. *Contraction duration depends on muscle fiber type (a), contractile force varies with muscle length (b), and velocity of contraction decreases as load increases (c).*

of muscles to their function. Ocular muscles (fiber II), which must cause extremely rapid movement of the eyes, contract more rapidly than almost any other muscle. The gastrocnemius muscle (fiber II + I) must contract moderately rapidly since it is used when jumping and performing rapid movements of the foot. The soleus (fiber I) does not need to contract rapidly because it is used principally for support of the body against gravity.

The force of muscle contraction strongly depends on the length to which the muscle is stretched before contraction is initiated (Fig. 2b): it contracts with maximum force when at its normal resting length. If the muscle is stretched to much greater than its normal length, the resting tension increases, thus decreasing the active tension (tension during contraction) . When the muscle is at less than normal length, the active tension also decreases. A muscle contracts very rapidly when it contracts against no load. However, when loads are applied, the velocity of contraction decreases (Fig.2c).

The muscle contraction force depends on the number of active motor units. It increases as the number of activated motor units increases (Fig. 3a). The force also depends on the number of successive action potentials and their spacing in time (wave summation). Wave summation occurs when each muscle fiber contracts in rapid succession—the contractions occurring closely enough so that a new contraction occurs before the previous one is over, thus adding its force to the preceding contraction. Tetanization is reached when muscle twitches become fused into a single prolonged contraction (Fig.3b). In general, natural skeletal muscle force control is achieved by varying the number of activated motor units and their rate of activation—the small motor units being activated first, the large one later (natural recruitment process).

Skeletal muscle contractions evoked by single action potentials are much different from those of cardiac muscles: in cardiac muscles the duration of contraction and refractory period are much longer and the wave summation phenomenon does not occur (Fig.3c).

Skeletal Muscle Electrical Stimulation[3,4]

Action potentials can be effected by subjecting a nerve to a rapidly changing electrical field. This phenomenon is known as electrical excitation, activation, or stimulation. An action potential so evoked is indistinguishable, by the end organ, from an action potential resulting from a natural control process.

An electrical charge artificially induced across the nerve membrane(e.g., with an electrode placed near the nerve fiber, Fig. 4a) causes an excess flow of ions through the membrane. At the electrode site (− cathode), the potential outside the membrane is made negative with respect to that of the inside. A weak cathodic potential cannot excite the fiber. However, when this potential is increased above threshold, excitation takes place. Further increase above threshold values does not change the nature of action potential (Fig.4b). One example of electrical pulses frequently used is shown in Figure 5. Biphasic cathodic pulses (b) are preferred to monophasic pulses (a) to minimize electrochemical damages at the electrode site (see later).

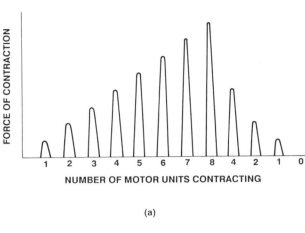

(a)

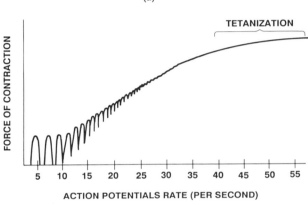

(b)

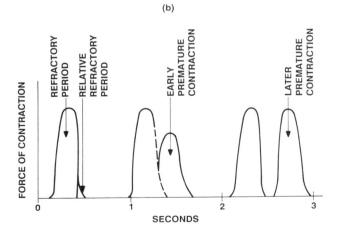

(c)

Figure 3. *Muscle force increases as more motor units are activated (a) and/or as the rate of action potential generation is increased (b). Contrary to skeletal muscle, cardiac muscle contraction lasts much longer and the wave summation process does not occur (c).*

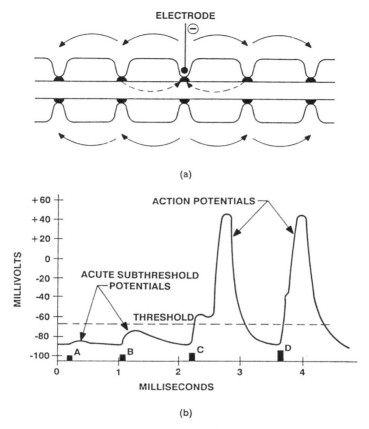

Figure 4. *Electrical stimulation of a myelinated axon (a) and resulting evoked action potential (b). As electrode potential is increased above threshold, axon excitation takes place.*

Response of a single myelinated fiber to electrical stimulation can be modeled[3] and depends on the following parameters:

a. *electrical:* the pulse amplitude required to evoke an action potential decreases as the pulse width increases (strength-duration curve, Fig. 6a). The efficacy of stimulation, as shown by the amount of charge (Cb) required for nerve excitation (product of pulse amplitude [A] by pulse width [s]), is higher with narrow pulses (e.g., narrow pulses require less charge to evoke action potential Fig. 6b).

b. *electrode position:* as the electrode to nerve distance increases, the threshold pulse amplitude increases (Fig. 7a).

c. *nerve fiber diameter:* due to their larger internodal distances, large fibers have a lower stimulation threshold than small fibers (Fig. 7b).

In practice, nerve fibers are not isolated and stimulation of nerve bundles

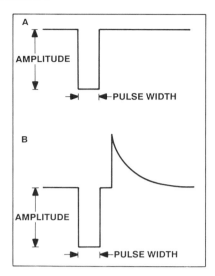

Figure 5. *Monophasic (a) and biphasic (b) electrical stimulation impulses.*

occurs. Bundles generally are composed of different axon diameters. A stimulus pulse at amplitude just above threshold will excite the closest and largest fibers. As the pulse amplitude (or pulse width) is increased, polarization of membranes will be sufficient to excite smaller fibers as well as fibers farther away.[2] This phenomenon is called "spatial recruitment."

The evoked muscle force can therefore be graded by varying either the pulse amplitude or the pulse width (Fig. 8). As amplitude (or pulse width) is increased, no muscle response is observed until threshold of the most excitable motor units is reached. Increase beyond supramaximal levels results in no additional increase in force.

Applying a succession of stimulation pulses enables a further increase of the evoked force and/or the ability to sustain it for a longer period of time (Fig. 9a). This phenomenon is called "temporal recruitment." As the interval between stimuli is shortened, the muscle does not return to its resting tension between responses. When the stimuli becomes sufficiently frequent, the summating contractions fuse and cannot be individually distinguished (tetanization). Response depends on muscle fiber type: slow-twitch fiber muscle will display a lower fusion frequency than fast-twitch fiber muscles (e.g. 10 Hz vs 50 Hz, respectively).

The rate at which muscle fatigues during sustained contraction is affected by the stimulation frequency. It also depends on muscle fiber type, its history (conditioning), and the duty cycle to which it is subjected (stimulation time vs rest time). Generally, minimizing the stimulation frequency (e.g., 20 Hz) minimizes fatigue (Fig. 9b).

The electrical excitability of skeletal muscle fibers is substantially lower (higher threshold) than that of motor nerves. The relationship is illustrated in Figure 10. At short pulse durations (<100 sec), direct muscle fiber stimu-

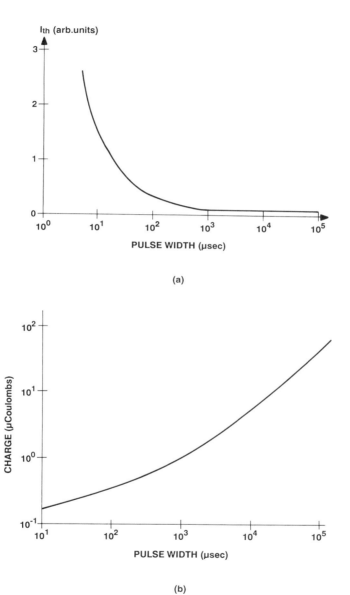

(a)

(b)

Figure 6. *Strength-duration curves for muscle stimulation via its nerve branches (a) and charge required versus stimulus pulse width (b).*

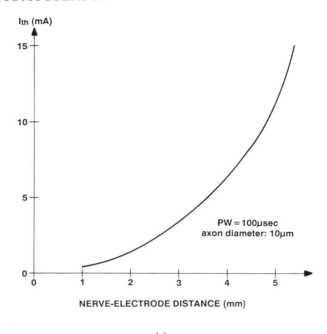

(a)

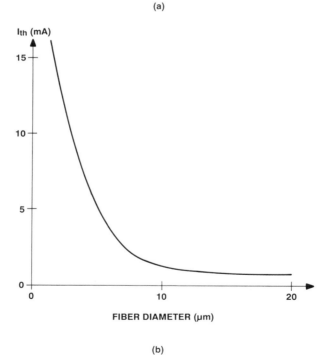

(b)

Figure 7. *Stimulus threshold dependence on nerve-electrode relative distance (a) and myelinated nerve fiber diameter (b).*

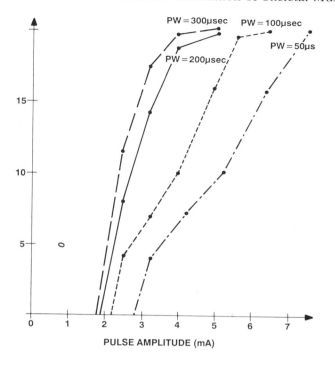

(a)

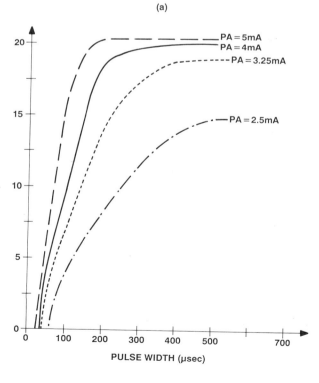

(b)

Figure 8. *Stimulus pulse amplitude (a) and pulse width (b) spatial recruitment curves.*

TEMPORAL RECRUITMENT

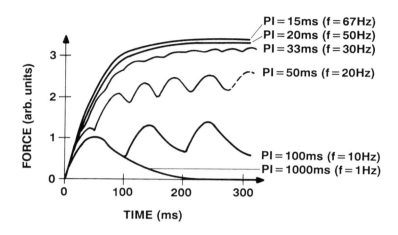

(a)

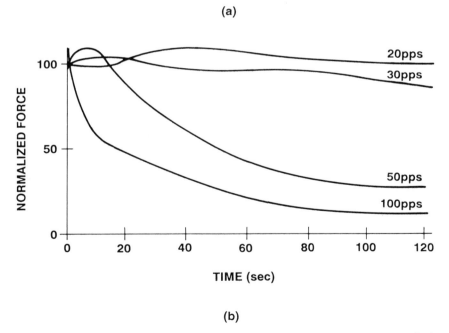

(b)

Figure 9. *Temporal recruitment (a) and muscle fatigue dependence on stimulation frequency (b).*

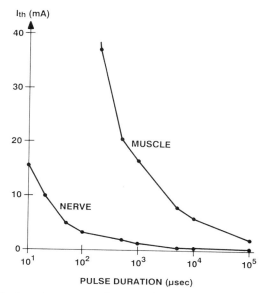

Figure 10. *Strength-duration curves for muscle stimulation via depolarization of its nerve or directly via its muscular fibers.*

lation requires a much greater stimulus amplitude than "indirect" muscle excitation (direct excitation of motor nerves). Increasing the pulse width reduces the pulse amplitude required. The energy required in the latter case however is very high and may jeopardize electrode electrochemical stability and be detrimental to neural tissues.

Recruitment of all the fibers of a denervated muscle is also a difficult task: since there is no spread of motor units, each muscle fiber needs to be depolarized individually. This may be very difficult to achieve in large muscles.

Electrodes for Skeletal Muscle Stimulation

To optimize their use, neuromuscular electrodes must be characterized with respect to their spatial recruitment characteristics, dependence on muscle length, stimulation energy and selectivity[5]:

a. recruitment length dependence is the change of spatial recruitment with muscle length variation
b. recruitment rate is the slope of evoked force versus pulse amplitude (or pulse width)
c. stimulation energy
d. selectivity of stimulation is an indication how localized or specific the stimulation is to a chosen muscle.

Such investigations must be performed for different electrode positions.

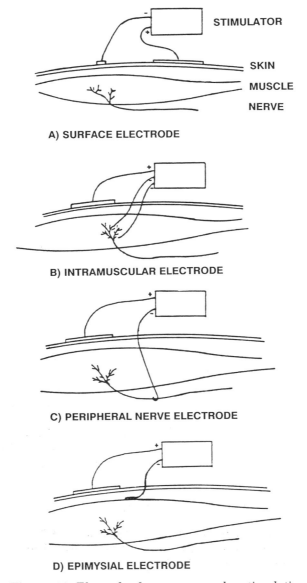

Figure 11. *Electrodes for neuromuscular stimulation.*

Neuromuscular electrodes can be classified into four main categories: surface, intramuscular, peripheral nerve, and epimysial electrodes (Fig. 11). Some spatial recruitment characteristics are reported in Figure 12.

a. surface electrodes: the anode and cathode are both placed on the skin surface; the cathode being over the nerve or muscle to be excited. The main disadvantage of such a system is its lack of selectivity of stimulation and

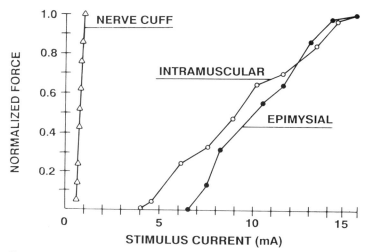

Figure 12. *Recruitment characteristics of nerve, intramuscular, and epimysial electrodes.*

repeatability since small movements of the cathode on the skin may cause large changes in muscle response. In addition, undesirable sensations (stimulation of sensory nerves) have been reported.

b. intramuscular electrodes: one or more are placed in the muscle body. Long-term stable and repeatable contractions can be achieved since the electrode is firmly positioned with respect to the nerve branches. Recruitment is gradual, but it may vary with muscle length. Biocompatibility of intramuscular electrodes shown in Figure 14 has been found to be very good.

c. peripheral nerve electrodes: the electrode is placed near or around the nerve controlling the desired muscle. Long-term stimulation can be achieved and the recruitment is independent of muscle length. The main disadvantage of such electrodes is the difficulty to grade the force developed by the muscle (all/none response). In addition, the surgery required may be very delicate and nerve damage may occur as the result of mechanical trauma rather than electrical stimulation.

Different nerve electrode types are shown in Figure 13. Cuff electrode (a) surrounds the nerve to localize current spread. Tight fit, although desirable, should be avoided to prevent nerve compression (e.g., in case of swelling) and irreversible nerve damage. Nerve electrode (b) is placed under the nerve and attached to surrounding tissues.[6] It does not prevent current to spread to surrounding tissues, but it decreases the risk of nerve compression.

The circumneural helical (c) electrode[7] and the spiral nerve cuff electrode (d)[8] are used to provide a snug fit around the nerve bundle without compressing the nerve.

d. epimysial electrode: the disk-shaped electrode (Fig. 14c) is sutured on the muscle epimysium, preferably in a high neural density area.[5,6] This minimizes the possibility of nerve injury and placement is atraumatic.

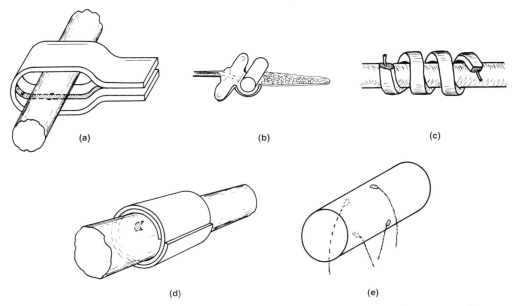

Figure 13. *Nerve electrode configurations. (a) full cuff, (b) semi-cuff,[7] (c) helical,[8] (d) spiral cuff,[20] and (e) multipolar.[9,10]*

Multipolar nerve electrodes (Fig. 13e) have been developed and investigated.[9,10] These designs aim at selectively recruiting specific nerve fibers within the nerve bundle. By selecting different poles, the potential exists to control muscle force in a finer way than is possible with a cuff electrode. In a similar way, multipolar cyclic stimulation may also decrease the occurrence of muscle fatigue.[9] It also creates the potential for selective stimulation of muscles innervated from a common nerve trunk. However, this requires long-term stability of electrode position with any movement.

Whatever the electrode type used, the application of an electrical field to neural tissues involves electron flow in the metal components and ion flow in the tissue medium. Conversion between the two processes occurs at the metal-tissue interface. Knowledge of the processes that occur at this interface is critical, but they are only partially known.[4] The electrode material, its surface characteristics as well as the excitation waveform are of the utmost importance.

Under passive conditions (no stimulus applied), thermodynamic forces bring the metal and ionic solution into equilibrium, resulting in an equilibrium potential. Inhomogeneities on the metal surface may produce local potential differences that may favor continued loss of metal ions (e.g., corrosion). Some metals or alloys have a greater tendency than others to exhibit this type of corrosion and therefore are less suitable for use as stimulating electrodes. Generally, the material of choice is platinum or platinum iridium alloys.

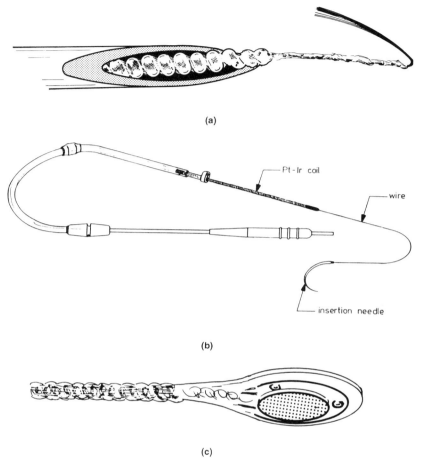

(a)

(b)

(c)

Figure 14. *(a) Percutaneous intramuscular electrodes,*[4] *(b) intramuscular electrode for permanent implant,*[1,19] *and (c) epimysial electrode.*[6]

The application of an external potential source to the electrode forces electron flow in the metal that alters the field distribution (from equilibrium) at the metal-solution interface. The altered charge distribution is reflected in the resting electrode potential that will vary more if the stimulus is large and the electrode surface is small (large charge density).

If the equilibrium potential is located in the reversible region, charge can be added to or subtracted from the metal surface in a reversible manner. Using biphasic pulses enable one to stay within this safe reversible region. Charges of 0.45 to 2 Cb/mm^2 have been reported to be safe with platinum electrodes.[4]

Great care is required in electrode material selection, manufacturing process, and handling since any of these factors may result in electrochemical electrode instability during stimulation.

Clinical Applications

Electrical stimulation of the nervous system makes it possible to externally control the motor system, thus providing the opportunity to restore impaired body functions. Some applications are reviewed below.

Correction of Footdrop in Hemiplegic Patients[11]

The system is designed to dorsiflex the ankle during the swing phase of gait by electrical stimulation of the peroneal nerve. An example of such a system (Fig. 15) is composed of the following: (1) an external stimulator and antenna that generate and transmit a radio-frequency signal through the skin, (2) a heel switch transmitter that triggers the stimulator, and (3) a surgically implanted receiver that receives the signal from the stimulator and converts it to a series of impulses applied to the motor branches of the peroneal nerve via a bipolar cuff electrode (Figure 15b). Some patients have been stimulated for more than 12 years without complication, while others have encountered progressive nerve damage.

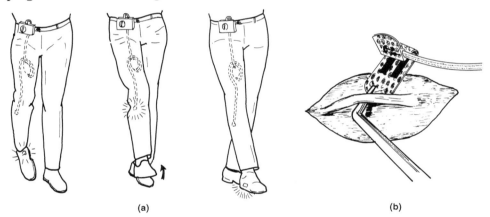

(a)   (b)

Figure 15. *Correction of footdrop in hemiplegic patient (a) and cuff electrode placement around nerve (b).*

Respiratory Assistance

Pulmonary dysfunction resulting from the loss of higher central nervous system control has been overcome in humans by electrical activation of the phrenic nerve. The stimulation systems used have been subcutaneous implants powered by radio frequency with leads attached to the phrenic nerve (Fig. 16a). Bilateral implants usually are used in quadriplegic patients. Activation of a single phrenic nerve provides adequate ventilation for 8–12 hours per 24-hour

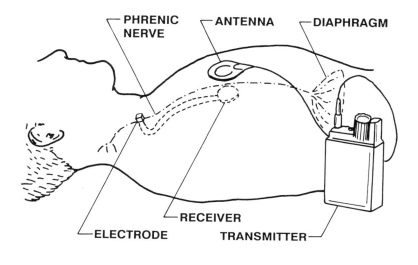

(a)

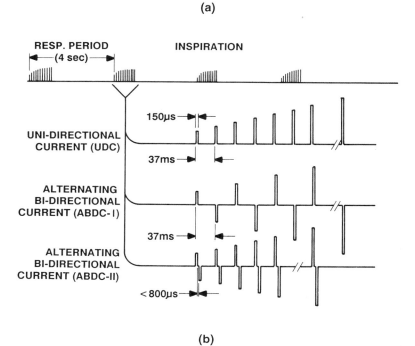

(b)

Figure 16. *System for respiration assistance by phrenic nerve stimulation (a) and stimulation paradigm (b).*

period. Longer periods of support can be achieved by stimulating one hemidiaphragm for a period of time and then the other.

The electrode systems employed have been bipolar, tripolar and more recently monopolar using different stimuli (Fig. 16b).[4,7] Some investigators have reported 24-hour ventilation support using quadripolar nerve electrodes with cyclic stimulation,[9] while others are investigating the use of intramuscular electrodes placed in the diaphragm by laparoscopic technique.[12]

Scoliosis Correction

Electrical activation of muscles acting on the spinal column in principle can apply a corrective force on the deformed, scoliotic spine. It offers the possibility of treating scoliosis in the growing child while avoiding the undesirable cosmetic effect of a brace. Systems investigated are either totally implantable (using muscle electrodes connected to implantable stimulator) or external (transcutaneous stimulation). Stimulation is applied during the sleeping period (e.g., 30 Hz, 1 sec on, 10 sec off).[4]

Upper Extremity Stimulation

Tetraplegic patients (C-6 level) retain voluntary control of elbow flexion and some control of forearm supination but have no control of wrist and hand function.

Palmar and lateral prehensions can be restored by multimuscle stimulation (Fig. 17). The system is composed of an external stimulator (8 channels), shoulder controller, an implantable receiver/stimulator, and electrodes. Finger movements are directed by the patient's shoulder controller (command signal). Adjustment is achieved mainly by visual feedback. Some sensory and auditory feedback signals have been added to enable better control. Intramuscular (Fig. 14a) and epimysial (Fig. 14c) electrodes have been used successfully in many patients. Force control is achieved by pulse width and pulse interval modulation. The major difficulty remains the absence of tactile feedback in these patients.[13]

Lower Extremity Stimulation

Complex electrical stimulation of lower extremities has enabled paraplegics to stand up, then "walk," and finally, to go up and down stairs. This is one of the most complex applications since muscle strength is required to keep the body in a standing position, while fine control is required to evoke gait patterns. Although balance remains a major problem, some patients have been able to walk at a rather high speed (1–1.5 m/sec) for up to 800 meters with the help of a walker.[14]

This approach requires multimuscle stimulation, and up to 48 channels of stimulation have been required to provide the gait pattern (Fig. 18). The

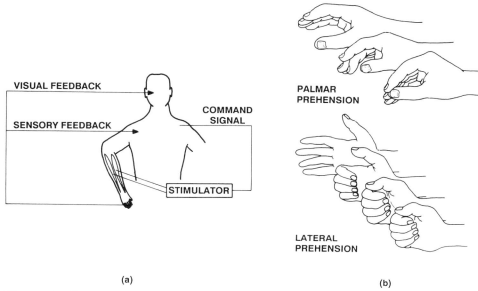

Figure 17. *Upper extremity control system for quadriplegics (a) and evoked grasp patterns (b).*

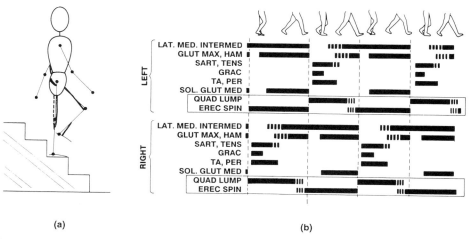

Figure 18. *Lower extremity control in paraplegics (a) and example of stimulation pattern to achieve coordinated leg movements (b).*

electrodes used in this situation are intramuscular (Fig. 14a), and muscle control is obtained by pulse width and pulse interval modulation.

Discussion

In the future, major improvements in electrical stimulation of skeletal muscles may result from a better understanding of basic muscle physiology and improved control systems (electrodes, stimulators, and sensors).[15]

Basic muscle research may elucidate the phenomenon by which muscles adapt to workloads and indicate the best way to use them efficiently. Bioengineering research may lead to better control of the stimulation of neural tissues. For instance, present electrodes evoke action potentials that propagate bidirectionally along nerve fibers. Recent papers have reported new electrode designs that generate unidirectional action potentials.[16]

Contrary to the natural process, electrical stimulation recruits large myelinated fibers first, then smaller fibers. Recent papers indicate that there are ways to reverse this recruitment order.[17]

Many applications may require a finer control of muscle contraction than presently achieved with open-loop systems. Closed-loop control with the addition of new sensors will be required to feed information back to the stimulator in a first stage and ultimately directly to the subject's own nervous system (Fig. 19).[18]

Experimental and clinical knowledge gathered in the wide field of functional electrical stimulation has been extremely useful in providing the basis

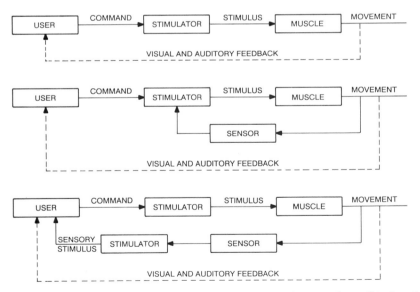

Figure 19. *Control configurations for muscle stimulation. (a) open loop, (b) closed-loop control with feedback to stimulator, and (c) closed-loop control with sensory feedback to patient.*[18]

for the development of techniques using skeletal muscles to assist heart function.[19] Additional knowledge and improved techniques developed for the various applications reviewed here, as well as for innovative future applications, improved communication between investigators, and exchange of basic, applied, and clinical information gained in the different application fields will provide the basis for a better understanding of phenomenon, which will result in improved clinical performance and patient benefit.

Acknowledgment: Special thanks to the following people for the information provided: J.T. Mortimer, J. Sweeney (Applied Neural Control Laboratory, Cleveland); R. Kobetic (Veterans Administration Hospital, Cleveland); D. McNeal, R. Waters (Rancho Rehabilitation Engineering Center, Downey); W.W.Glenn (Yale University); H. Peckham (MetroHealth Hospital, Cleveland); W.F. Agnew (Huntington Medical Research Institutes, Pasadena), and J. de Jonge for assistance with illustrations.

References

1. Carpentier A, Chachques JC: Myocardial substitution with a stimulated skeletal muscle: first successful clinical case. Lancet 8440:1267, 1985.
2. Guyton AC: Textbook of Medical Physiology. Philadelphia, WB Saunders, 1980, pp 106–148.
3. Benton LA, LL Baker, BR Bolman, et al: Functional Electrical Stimulation—A Practical Clinical Guide. Rancho los Amigos Hospital, Downey, CA, 1981.
4. Mortimer JT: Motor Prostheses. In VB Brooks (ed): Handbook of Physiology: The Nervous System. Bethesda, American Physiological Society, 1981, pp 155–187.
5. Grandjean PA: Recruitment properties of subfascial monopolar and bipolar electrodes. Master Thesis Case Western Reserve University, Cleveland, 1983.
6. Grandjean PA, JT Mortimer: Recruitment properties of epimysial electrodes. Ann Biomed Eng, 14:53, 1986.
7. Glenn WW: Diaphragm pacing by electrical stimulation of the phrenic nerve. Neurosurgery 17:974, 1985.
8. Agnew WF, McCreery DB, Yuen TGH, et al: Histologic and physiologic evaluation of electrically stimulated peripheral nerve: consideration of selection of parameters. Ann Biomed Eng 17:39, 1989.
9. Thoma H: Functional electrostimulation: basics, technology and applications. lst Vienna Workshop Proceedings, Oct. 1983.
10. McNeal DR, Bowman BR: Selective activation of muscle using peripheral nerve electrodes. Med Biol Eng Comput 23:249, 1985.
11. McNeal DR, Waters RL: Rehabilitation Engineering Center Grant on Functional Electrical Stimulation: Reports of Progress 1988.
12. Nochomovitz M: Electrical activation of respiration. Eng Med Bio June:25, 1983.
13. Peckham PH, Marsolais EB, Mortimer JT: Restoration of key grip and release in the C6 tetraplegic patient through functional electrical stimulation. J Hand Surg 5:5, 1980.
14. Marsolais EB, Kobetic R: 4th Annual Applied Neural Control Research Day. Case Western Reserve University, Cleveland. May 1989.
15. Crago PE, Chizek HJ, Neuman MR, et al: Sensors for use with functional neuromuscular stimulation. IEEE Trans Biomed Eng 33:256, 1986.
16. Sweeney JD, Mortimer JT: An asymetric two electrode cuff for generation of unidirectionally propagated action potentials. IEEE Trans Biomed Engr 33:541, 1986.
17. Fang ZP, Mortimer JT: A method for attaining natural recruitment order in artificially activated muscles. Proceedings 9th Annual Conference IEEE Eng Med Biol Soc, pp 657–658, 1987.

18. Cybulski GR, Penn RD, Jaeger RJ: Lower extremity functional electrical stimulation in cases of spinal cord injury. Neurosurgery 15:1, 1984.
19. Chiu R C-J: Biomechanical Cardiac Assist: Cardiomyoplasty and Muscle-Powered Devices. Mount Kisco, NY, Futura Publishing Company, 1986.
20. Naples GG, Mortimer JT, Scheiner A, et al: A spiral nerve cuff electrode for peripheral nerve stimulation. IEEE Trans Biomed Eng 35:905, 1988.

Chapter 5

Anatomy of the Latissimus Dorsi Muscle

I. Description
Patrick Perier, Christophe Acar,
Juan-Carlos Chachques

II. Segmental Anatomy and Function
Olav M. Sola, B.A. Kakulas, Robert Thomas

III. Intramuscular Vascularization
Marc A. Radermecker, Jacques Fourny,
J. Fissette, Raymond Limet

I. Description

Intrathoracic muscle transposition was first described in 1911 by Abrashanoff as a mean to close a bronchopleural fistula.[1] In recent years, a considerable amount of interest has been generated by the widespread use of the pedicled latissimus dorsi myocutaneous and muscle flaps in plastic and reconstructive surgery.[2-5] In addition, there has been increasing interest in the use of this muscle flap for reconstructive cardiac surgery.[6-8]

The anatomy of the muscle and the specific size, pattern, and location of the primary neurovascular pedicle are important considerations when this muscle is used for cardiac reconstruction.

Gross Muscle Anatomy

The latissimus dorsi is a broad, flat triangular muscle that covers the lumbar and lower half of the dorsal region with a narrow fasciculus at its insertion on the humerus.[9,10] Multiple tendinous fibers arise from the spinous

From *Cardiomyoplasty* edited by Alain Carpentier, MD, PhD, Juan-Carlos Chachques, MD, and Pierre Grandjean, MS © 1991. Futura Publishing Inc., Mount Kisco, NY.

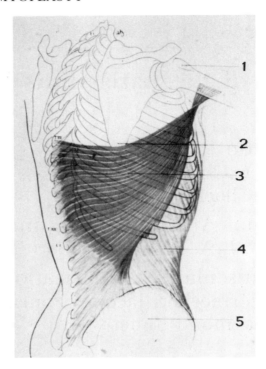

Figure 1. *Insertions of latissimus dorsi. 1 = humerus; 2 = scapula; 3 = latissimus dorsi; 4 = external oblique; 5 = ilium.*

processes of the six or seven inferior dorsal vertebrae and from the posterior layer of the lumbar fascia (Fig. 1). Tendinous fibers also arise from the external lip of the crest of the ilium behind the origin of the external oblique. Fleshy digitations are attached on the three or four lower ribs that are interposed between similar processes of the external oblique muscle.

From this extensive origin, the fibers pass in different directions: the upper ones horizontally, the middle obliquely upward, and the lower vertically upward. These fibers converge and form a thick fasciculus that crosses the inferior angle of the scapula and occasionally receives a few fibers from it.

The muscle then curves around the lower border of the teres major and is twisted upon itself so that the superior fibers become at first posterior and then inferior and the vertical fibers at first anterior and then superior. It then terminates in a short quadrilateral tendon about three inches in length that, passing in front of the tendon of the teres major, is inserted into the bottom of the bicipital groove of the humerus. This insertion extends higher on the humerus than that of the tendon of the pectoralis major. The lower border of the tendon of this muscle is united with that of the teres major.

The superficial surface of the latissimus dorsi is subcutaneous, except in its upper part, where it is partially covered with the trapezius and at its insertion where its tendon is crossed by the axillary vessels and the brachial plexus of nerves.

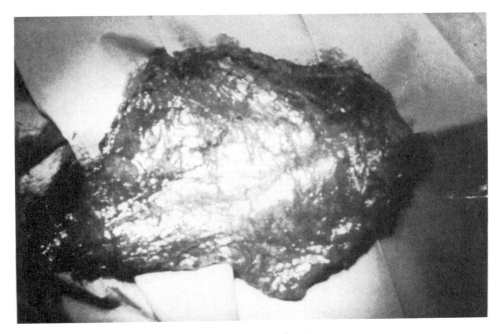

Figure 2. *Aspect of a flap.*

The deep surface is in contact with the lumbar fascia, the serratus posticus inferior, the lower external intercostal muscles and ribs, inferior angle of the scapula, rhomboid major, infraspinous, and teres major. Its outer margin is separated below from the external oblique by a small triangular interval, the triangle of Petit.

The latissimus dorsi draws the arm medially and posteriorly as it rolls the arm inward in an adduction positi. The muscle also pulls the scapula in a medial and downward direction.

Anthropometric Anatomical Study

Anthropometric studies were performed on the left latissimus dorsi muscle in ten human cadavers (5 females and 5 males) (Fig. 2).[11] The study included: (1) measurement of the length of the anterior and posterior borders of the muscle and the length of the muscle at its middle portion; (2) measurement of the width of the muscle at the level of its upper, middle, and lower parts; (3) measurement of the thickness of the muscle anteriorly, medially, and posteriorly. The results are shown in Table 1.

Vascularization

The primary vascular supply of the latissimus dorsi is the thoracodorsal artery and vein. These vessels are branches of the subscapular artery and vein that originate from the axillary artery and vein, respectively (Fig. 3).[9,10]

Table 1
Anatomical Dimensions of the Latissimus Dorsi
Expressed in Centimeters ± SED

Male					
Length		*Width*		*Thickness*	
Anteriorly	40 ± 2.2	Upper part	7.2 ± 0.8	Anteriorly	1.22 ± 0.13
Middle part	36 ± 2.0	Middle part	13.4 ± 2.9	Middle part	1.22 ± 0.19
Posteriorly	32 ± 2.1	Lower part	33.4 ± 3.3	Posteriorly	0.94 ± 0.05
Female					
Anteriorly	38 ± 2.8	Upper part	6.6 ± 1.1	Anteriorly	1.26 ± 0.08
Middle part	34 ± 3.1	Middle part	11.4 ± 2.1	Middle part	1.14 ± 0.19
Posteriorly	33 ± 3.2	Lower part	30.6 ± 4.3	Posteriorly	1.02 ± 0.16

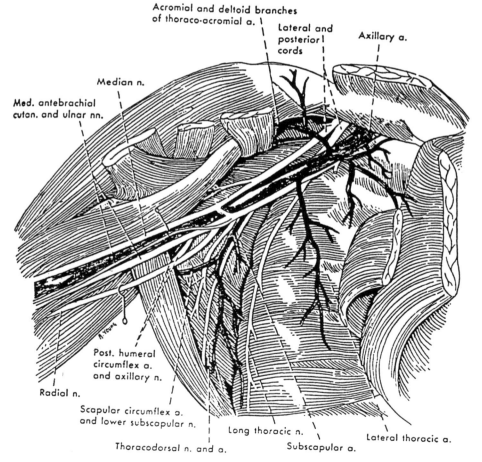

Figure 3. *Vascularization and innervation of the latissimus dorsi.*

Subscapular and Circumflex Scapular Vascular Anatomy

In 92% of the cases studied by Bartlett et al.,[12] the subscapular artery and vein in close contact originated from the axillary artery and vein. In 8%, the artery and the vein were separated at their origin, a distance of 4.2 cm from each other, and joined together 5.6 cm more distally.

The subscapular artery and vein then bifurcate into circumflex scapular vessels and thoracodorsal vessels. Although rare, variations have been observed[12]: the circumflex artery or vein can arise directly from the axillary vessels or double circumflex arteries or veins may be observed. In a few cases small arterial branches from the subscapular artery are present before its major bifurcation into the circumflex scapular and thoracodorsal arteries.

Thoracodorsal Artery and Vein

The blood supply to the latissimus dorsi essentially comes from the thoracodorsal artery and vein.

The artery may gives rise to one, two, or three branches to the chest wall before entering the latissimus dorsi. The mean length of thoracodorsal vessels is 9.3 mm (6.0 mm to 16.5 mm) and the mean diameter of the artery is 2.7 mm (range 1.5–4.0 mm) at origin and 1.6 mm (range 0.5–3.5 mm) at the neurovascular hilus of latissimus dorsi.[12]

It is important to note that the suprascapular vein and the origin of the thoracodorsal vein do have valves.

The Neurovascular Hilum

The thoracodorsal artery and vein enter the inferior surface of the latissimus dorsi at a clearly defined neurovascular hilum, usually single. Occasionally two hila can be observed. The mean location of the hilum is 8.7 ± 0.14 cm distal to the subscapular artery origin (range 6.0–11.5 cm) and 2.6 ± 0.07 cm medial to the lateral border of the muscle (range 1–4 cm).[13] Division of the thoracodorsal artery uniformly occurs at the neuvascular hilum.

The pattern of major branching of the thoracodorsal artery and vein is a bifurcation. The upper or medial vessels course transversely across the muscle parallel to the superior border 3.5 cm from the edge and separate from the lower or lateral vessels at the neurovascular hilum at a 45° angle.

The lateral vessel is usually the larger and its course parallels the lateral border of the muscle at a mean distance of 2.1 cm towards the iliac crest. Within the substance of the distal muscle, the lateral branch gives rise to one or more large branches that course parallel to the medial branch and the distal muscle fibers. In some cases, the neurovascular tree arborizes into three or four major branches that course parallel to each other and the distal muscle fibers.

Secondary Vascular Supply

Secondary vascular supplies representing distal vascular pedicles from posterior intercostal vessels exist and can support the flap entirely when the primary vascular pedicle is interrupted.[14]

Neural Anatomy

The innervation of the latissimus dorsi is through the thoracodorsal nerve derived from the posterior cord of the brachial plexus,[9,10] originating from the sixth, seventh, and eighth cervical vertebrae. The nerve can be seen at a mean distance of 3.1 cm proximal to the subscapular artery and vein, joining them within 3 to 9 cm, and paralleling the vasculature to the neurovascular hilum of the latissimus dorsi muscle. At the neurovascular hilus, the branching pattern of the nerve parallels that of the vasculature.

As a result of its more lengthy proximal portion, the thoracodorsal nerve is somewhat longer than its venous and arterial counterpart — a mean length of 12.3 cm with a range of 8.5 cm to 19 cm.

Conclusion

The size and the length of the primary vascular pedicle make the latissimus dorsi an ideal flap. It should be noted that the branching of both the neural and vascular supplies of the latissimus dorsi muscle occurs at a consistent proximally located site near the flap rotation point. It is also of interest that the neurovascular branching patterns within the muscle substance also are consistent with little significant variation and provide the medial and lateral portions of the muscle within independent neurovascular supplies.

II. Segmental Anatomy and Function

Growing interest in the use of the latissimus dorsi (LD) by plastic surgeons and more recently by cardiac surgeons motivated us to review the segmental anatomy and function of this muscle. Our study was carried out in human cadavers and living dogs.

Dissection

Following removal of skin and subcutaneous fat, the external surface of the LD was found to be covered with a strong, tough layer of fibro-fatty tissue, the external fascia. Attempts to dissect through this layer led to tearing of muscle and disruption of its architecture, particularly in human specimens. Another approach was then developed. The lower end of the trapezius was freed and lifted cephalad. An incision was made medial to the tip of the scapula and extended laterally and posteriorly. Dissection of the LD muscle from the aponeurosis of the spinal processes of T-6 through T-12 was performed carefully. Special care had to be taken inferiorly because the serratus posterior inferior originate from the deep portion of the aponeurosis, extends laterally and, is intimately associated with the LD muscle. The origins in the lumbodorsal fascia and intercostal sites were freed, along with numerous interdigitations to the underlying structures. The freed tendinous insertion was a long, narrow structure that gave the appearance of rotation prior to insertion into the intertubercular groove in the humerus. In the dog, the structure, which corresponds to the tendon in the human LD muscle, is distinctive. It does not insert into the humerus; rather it has a notched ending that encircles the humerus in a diffuce manner that is destroyed easily during dissection.

Segments

Upon removal of the muscle from both human and canine sources, the internal or deep surface was found to be covered with a thin, flimsy areolar fascia. Removal of this fascia revealed three distinct segments: the transverse, oblique, and lateral segments.

The transverse and lateral segments form a stylized figure of 7 (Fig. 4). In humans, the angle of these two segments varies between 45° and 90°, depending on the individual.

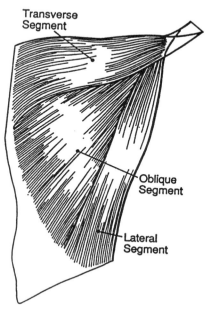

Figure 4. *In both humans and canines, the deep surface of the LD muscle shows three distinct segments with fibers oriented in transverse, oblique, and lateral directions.*

The transverse segment arises from the aponeurosis of the spinal processes of T-6 through T-9 and extends laterally and superiorly beneath the tip of the scapula, often fusing with the teres major, and rotates inferiorly to form the lower portion of the tendon. The thickness of this segment can vary considerably.

The oblique segment arises from the thoracodorsal aponeurosis of T-9 through T-12 and extends obliquely upward at 45°. The fascicles can be isolated as wide, thin, flat structures extending from the aponeurosis to the tendon.

The lateral segment arises from the lower two ribs and the lumbodorsal fascia. It varies from 25–35 cm in length and 5–7 cm in width. The fibers are symmetrical, fascicles overlap posteriorly, and the segment extends superiorly at 10°-30° from the vertebral column. The fibers narrow to form the posterior superior portion of the tendon, inserting into the groove of the humerus.

Function

It is useful to think of the LD as three distinct muscles or segments, each contracting in a different direction, allowing a wide range of movement of the upper extremity. Electromyographic studies of the transverse and lateral segments confirm the segmental activity (Fig. 5). Conversely, the lateral segment shows marked electrical activity during contraction related to downward movement of the extended arm. The oblique segment is a transition zone between transverse and lateral segments.

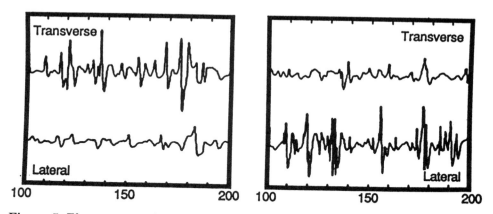

Figure 5. *Electromyographic study (left panel) shows activity in the transverse segment while the lateral segment is at rest during posterior refraction of the extended upper extremity. Electromyographic study (right panel) shows activity in the lateral segment while the transverse segment is at rest during downward motion of the laterally extended upper extremity.*

Blood Supply

Not only are the anatomy and function of the three segments different, the blood supply is also different. For the lateral segment it arises from the long anterior branch of the thoracodorsal artery that has several loop anastomoses. In contrast, the transverse and oblique segments are supplied by perforating thoracic, and intercostal vessels in addition to branches of the thoracodorsal artery.

Comparison of Human and Canine LD Muscle

Important differences exist between canine and human LD muscle. In canines, the LD is symmetrical in size, shape, and weight; is relatively longer; and tends to be consistent in thickness throughout the muscle. In 90% of human subjects, however, there is a marked variability both within subjects and between subjects. In most cases, the weight of the right LD muscle in humans was approximately 22% more on average than the left, in some instances, was up to 100% greater. Dissection of the canine LD is relatively easy. In the human, numerous fascial attachments and interdigitations are present, particularly with teres major and the posterior serratus inferior, making dissection of human LD difficult.

Conclusions

Because of differences in direction of the fibers of the various segments, the specialized segmental activity (particularly transverse and lateral), differences in blood supply, and difficulty in dissecting the transverse and oblique segments, we recommend that insofar as possible, the lateral segment of the LD should be used for cardiomyoplasty procedures.

III. Intramuscular Vascularization

Cardiomyoplasty, as described by Carpentier and Chachques,[6,7] uses skeletal striated muscle for three major purposes: reinforcement and support of the failing heart, substitution after myocardial wall resection, and reconstructive procedure for therapy of congenital cardiopathies. Although the use of several other muscle flaps has been advocated, latissimus dorsi seems to be the most suitable for these purposes. This technique requires preconditioning to transform a fast-twitch fatigable muscle into a slow-twitch fatigue-resistant one. This conditioning is accomplished by implanted stimulating electrodes that will allow later synchronous pacing of the heart's electrical activity.

This surgical technique requires peripheral dissection of the muscle flap with interruption of the peripheral vascularization and intramuscular positioning of stimulating electrodes. We therefore studied the intramuscular vascularization of the latissimus dorsi muscle so as to assess whether the thoracodorsalis artery can assume the blood supply for the distal portion of the muscle and whether the intramuscular electrodes compromise vascularization.

Materials and Methods

Fifteen human LD were carefully dissected in 15 fresh cadavers (8 male, 7 female). Anatomical macroscopic study of the subscapularis artery, circumflex artery, and thoracodorsalis artery was realized. Latissimus dorsi distal and peripheral muscular insertion and blood supplies (from intercostales and lumbaris arteries) were dissected and the anatomical piece was removed "en bloc," with careful preservation of the neurovascular pedicle. Anatomical details of thoracodorsalis artery division and nerve branches were studied. The intramuscular vascularization was highlighted by injection of the previously cannulated thoracodorsalis artery. Iodine radiocontrast was used. Analysis of the angiographic data was realized by radiologists and surgeons (Fig. 6).

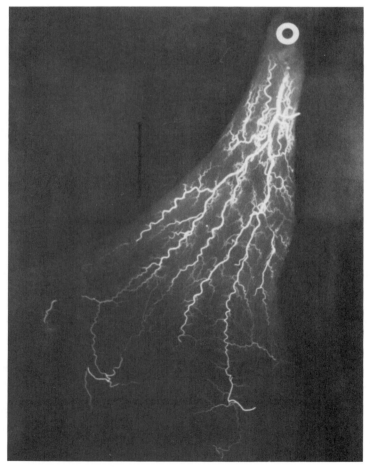

Figure 6. *Angiography of LD intramuscular vascularization through isolated thoracodorsalis artery contrast perfusion.*

Results

Subscapularis artery was found to arise 3 to 4 cm outside the acromiothoracic artery on the axillary artery. It quickly (2–6 cm) divides in two main branches: the circumflex scapulae artery that exits backward in spatium axillare mediale, and the thoracodorsalis artery. Only once did we note two circumflex scapulae arteries arising from the subscapularis artery. The thoracodorsalis artery is accompanied by one or two veins and is quickly reached by the latissimus dorsi nerve that comes from the inside. The thoracodorsalis artery follows the external edge of the latissimus dorsi (1–2 cm inside) and spreads on its internal surface. The artery gives one to three branches for the serratus anterior and then divides for the muscle itself.

The splitting of thoracodorsalis artery for LD is not consistent, occurring either within the muscle itself or up to 4 cm before the muscle. Unlike data previously reported in the literature, [10] we found that division in three main trunks occurs in 10/13 (66%) (Fig. 7A). In 50% of these cases, one of the three branches was a recurrent artery that goes upward to supply the vascularization of the proximal segment of the muscle (Fig. 7B). When this artery did not exist, vascularization was achieved through small recurrent branches from the main division trunks of thoracodorsalis artery. If one excludes these recurrent arteries, the vascularization of the distal part of the muscle was achieved in 66% by two main division branches and in 33% by three main division branches (Fig. 7).

The most external branch was always the most important in size. In four cases, there was evidence of a collateral from this branch to the serratus an-

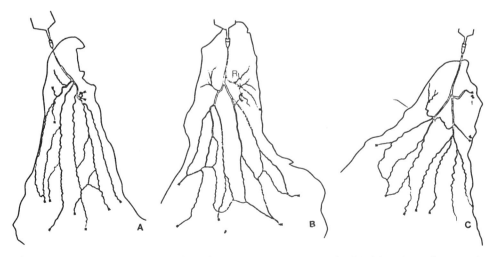

Figure 7. *Division of thoracodorsalis artery—variations. A. Division into three main branches, all distal. B. Division of thoracodorsalis artery in three main branches. One of the branches (R) is a recurrent artery. C. Division of thoracodorsalis artery into two main branches.*

		Table 2.			
L.D. Flap Number	No. of Major Bifurcation Trunks of T.D. Artery	Preponderance of the External Main Trunk		LB^x	DA^x
1	2	+		5	5
2	2	+		8	3
3	$3 (1 = R)^x$	+		5	2
4	2	+		5	4
5	3	+		9	5
6	$3 (1 = R)^x$	+		6	4
7	2	+		6	3
8	3	+		6	5
9	2	+		7	6
10	3	+		5	3
11	3	+		5	5
12	$3 (1 = R)^x$	+		6	4
13	$3 (1 = R)^x$	+		6	5
14	3	+		6	5
15	$3 (1 = R)^x$	+		6	5

LB = longitudinal intramuscular branches; DA = number of distal anastomoses with irrigation from lumbaris and intercostales arteries; (1 = R) = one of the three main trunks is a recurrent artery.

terior. These two or three major branches then divide into five to nine longitudinal arteries that go straight and progressively deeper to the distal part of the muscle where they anastomose with perforating arteries coming from intercostales and lumbaris arteries (Table 2). Angiographic data showed a sufficient distal blood supply as a result of thoracodorsalis artery selective perfusion.

Retrograde bleeding from unligated peripheral accessory supply was obvious. Major division branches of thoracodorsalis artery were accompanied by at least one division branch of latissimus dorsi nerves and veins. These neurovascular structures were situated in fatty cellular space between muscular fibrous bundles. Their pathway was easily visualized by gentle traction on the pedicle or careful dissection. As these structures progress distally, they ramify and penetrate deeper into the muscle.

Discussion and Conclusion

Although this angiological study is not always in agreement with previously published results from Bartlett et al.,[12] it establishes the constancy of the neurovascular pedicle and the intramuscular blood supply. We have shown that the intramuscular blood vascularization is achieved through 5 to 9 main longitudinal arteries that arise from the 2 or 3 main division branches of thoracodorsalis artery. Because of angiological evidence that thoracodorsalis blood supply anastomoses distally with peripheral vascularization from intercostales and lumbaris arteries, suppression of this vascularization during dissection of the muscle flap can be accomplished without fear of ischemic injury. This assessment is of primary importance when the aim of the flap mobilization is to obtain a biological endogenous energy source that will be used to assist a failing heart or to substitute a contracting myocardial wall.

For the purpose of cardiomyoplasty, the long-term stimulation of the skeletal muscle that will result in sustained fatigueless contraction is best obtained by depolarization of the intact motor nerve rather than by direct stimulation of the muscle fibers.[11]

To obtain muscle stimulation via its nerves, following the technique described by Carpentier, Chachques, and Grandjean, two electrodes are sewn into the muscle thickness. This procedure can theoretically injure the muscle vascularization and innervation. We noticed, however, that the superficial spreading of main division trunks and longitudinal arteries and their location in fatty cellular spaces made it possible to sew transversally two longitudinal electrode into the muscle without major injury to the blood supply of the flap.

We conclude that even through exclusive irrigation by thoracodorsalis artery there is a satisfying distal perfusion of the flap and that a minimal understanding of the intramuscular vascularization can preserve the muscle flap from neurovascular damage during surgical procedure.

References

1. Abrashanoff O: Plastiche methode der Schiessung von Fistelganger, welche von inneren Organen kommen. Zentralbl Chir 38:186, 1911.
2. Mutilbaner W, Olbrisch R: The latissimus dorsi myocutaneous flap for breast reconstruction. Chir Plastica 4:27, 1927.
3. Bostwick J, Vasconez LO, Jurkiewicz MJ: Breast reconstruction after a radical mastectomy. Plast Reconst Surg 61:682, 1978.
4. Quillen CG, Shearin JC, Georgiade NG: Use of the latissimus dorsi myocutaneous island flap for reconstruction of the head and neck area. Plast Reconst Surg 62:113, 1978.
5. Pairolero PC, Arnold PG, Piehler JM: Intrathoracic transposition of extrathoracic skeletal muscle. J Thorac Cardiovasc Surg 86:809, 1983.
6. Carpentier A, Chachques JC: Myocardial substitution with a stimulated skeletal muscle: first successful clinical case. Lancet 8440:1267, 1985.
7. Chachques JC, Grandjean P, Carpentier A: Dynamic cardiomyoplasty: experimental cardiac wall replacement with a stimulated muscle. In RC-J Chiu (ed): Biomechanical Cardiac Assist: Cardiomyoplasty and Muscle-Powered Devices. Mount Kisco, NY, Futura Publishing Co., 1986, p 59.
8. Carpentier A, Chachques JC: The use of stimulated skeletal muscle to replace disease human heart muscle. In RC-J Chiu (ed): Biomechanical Cardiac Assist: Cardiomyoplasty and Muscle-Powered Devices. Mount Kisco, NY, Futura Publishing Co., 1986, p 85.
9. Hollinsher WH: Textbook of Anatomy, 2nd ed. New York, Harper and Row, 1987, pp 200–201.
10. Gray: Anatomy, Descriptive and Surgical. New York, Bounty Books, 1977, pp 339–340.
11. Chachques JC, Grandjean P, Perier P, et al: Cardiomyoplastie. Bases expérimentales, technique opératoire, indications. Arch Mal Coeur 82:919, 1989.

12. Bartlett SP, May JW, Yaremchuk MJ: The latissimus dorsi muscle: a fresh cadaver study of the primary neurovascular pedicle. Plast Reconst Surg 67:631, 1981.
13. Tobin GR, Schusterman M, Peterson GH, et al: The intramuscular neurovascular anatomy of the latissimus dorsi muscle: the basis for splitting the flap. Plast Reconst Surg 67:637, 1982.
14. Tobin GR, Mavroudis C, Howe WR, et al: Reconstruction of complex thoracic defects with myocutaneous and muscle flaps.J Thorac Cardiovasc Surg 85:219, 1983.

Chapter 6

Experimental Basis of Cardiomyoplasty

Juan-Carlos Chachques, Alain Carpentier

The purpose of this chapter is to review preliminary works and experimental studies that have preceded the early clinical experience with cardiomyoplasty at Broussais Hospital. These studies were initiated in 1981 with the aim of resolving the specific problems raised by the wrapping of a skeletal muscle around the heart for long-term circulatory assistance, i.e., selection of the muscle, muscle conditioning, heart wrapping, and evaluation of performance.

Selection of the Muscle

Early attempts in other laboratories used either pectoralis muscle grafts or diaphragmatic pedicled grafts in dogs.[1,2] The latissimus dorsi was also used as an alternative by various authors because of its unique neurovascular pedicle and the possibility of its transfer into the thorax.[3] Electrostimulation of these muscles introduced the concept of cardiac assistance.[4-6] Preliminary studies in our laboratory, which will be summarized here, comprised anatomical investigation in human cadavers and experiments in dogs.[7]

In 10 human cadavers (5 males and 5 females), the left and right latissimus dorsi were dissected and measurements of length, width, and thickness of each flap were carried out. The average muscle thickness was 13 ± 2 mm near its origin and 10 ± 1.5 mm distally. Transfer of these flaps into the thorax after removing the anterior part of the second rib showed that each latissimus dorsi muscle flap could cover 100% of the homolateral ventricle and $70\% \pm 7\%$ of the contralateral ventricle in normal-sized hearts. In addition, each latissimus dorsi muscle flap could cover 100% of the homolateral atrium.

Acute experiments in dogs confirmed the feasibility of this operation in living animals (Fig. 1). It also allowed a comparison of the thresholds of electrical stimulation of denervated and contralateral nondenervated muscles. A

From *Cardiomyoplasty* edited by Alain Carpentier, MD, PhD, Juan-Carlos Chachques, MD, and Pierre Grandjean, MS © 1991. Futura Publishing Inc., Mount Kisco, NY.

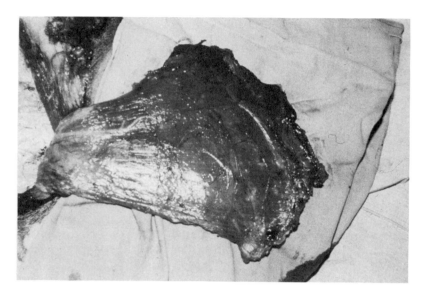

Figure 1A. *Latissimus dorsi muscle flap (LDMF).*

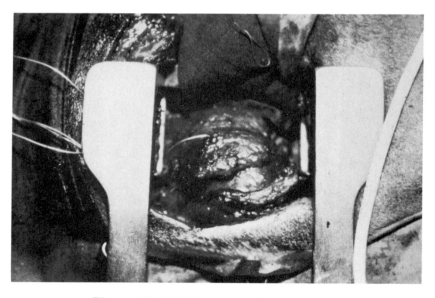

Figure 1B. *LDMF transposed over the heart.*

Pulse Width (ms)	Thresholds (mA)		
	Intact Muscle	Transposed Muscle	Denervated Muscle
0.2	0.9	2.5	6
0.4	0.9	2.5	5.6
0.6	0.7	2.5	5.2
0.8	0.5	2.3	4.4
1	0.5	2.4	4.4
1.2	0.5	2	4.2
1.4	0.4	2	4.2
1.6	0.4	2.1	4.2
1.8	0.4	2	4
2	0.4	2.1	4

Table 1

Different thresholds of stimulation expressed in milliamperes (mA) for intact muscle, transposed muscle over the heart (6-month follow-up), and denervated control latissimus dorsi muscles (6-month follow-up). Results were obtained for 10 pulse width values expressed in millisecond (msec).

striking difference was found when the thresholds were more than 2 times higher in denervated muscle than in nondenervated muscle (Table 1), thus ruling out the possibility of using a skeletal muscle as a denervated revascularized free flap.

Muscle Conditioning

Fatigue of the muscle and histochemical deleterious changes whenever a long-term stimulation was used had been stumbling blocks for many years in all institutions including our own.[6–8] The introduction of the concept of progressive sequential stimulation[9] overcame this problem and led to the development of a specific Cardiomyostimulator™ Pulse Train Generator. Experiments were carried out in goats.[10]

Material

Eleven alpine goats were operated for chronic long-term stimulation of the muscle. Latissimus dorsi muscles of five animals (group I) were stimulated with single pulses by means of intramuscular electrodes at pacing rates increasing gradually from 30 to 80 contractions per minute (10 ppm steps) every two weeks while latissimus dorsi muscles of another group of six animals (group II) were stimulated with bursts of pulses generated by programmable neuromuscular stimulators coupled to platinum-iridium (Pt/Ir) intramuscular electrodes. The number of bursts per minute were gradually increased from 30 to 80 (10 bpm steps) every 2 weeks, while preserving a duty cycle: T(ON)/ T(ON) + T(OFF) of 25%. Bursts were composed of 210-μs balanced charge cathodic pulses occurring at a frequency of 30 Hz. After a 2-year stimulation in group I and a 6-month stimulation in group II, electrophysiological and histochemical studies of the paced muscles and their contralaterals were carried out.

Electrophysiological Study

Two years in group I and 6 months in group II after stimulation, the medium and distal parts of the latissimus dorsi muscle were exposed and kept at fixed muscle length by upper-limb immobilization. A U-shaped semiconductor strain gauge was placed on the surface of the muscle parallel to its fibers to measure evoked forces and connected, via an analog, to a digital interface of an IBM portable computer. Evoked forces were stored in computer files for further analysis. Since muscle vascular and innervation supplies were preserved, this measurement technique enabled nondestructive investigation of unimpaired muscles.

Electrode recruitment characteristics (evoked force vs pulse amplitude) and electrode impedance were first measured with single pulse stimuli. Then forces evoked by bursts of impulses of fixed amplitude (maximum recruitment) were recorded. Burst durations were set to 1.5 sec and rest times at 4 sec. Frequency content varied from 2 to 85 Hz. These measurements enabled the determination of the fusion frequency, contraction time, and force dependence on burst frequency (temporal summation). Fatigue resistance was evaluated by measuring the decrease in evoked force over time (15 min) with muscles being paced with 250 ms ON, 750 ms OFF, 30 Hz pulse trains. Force was always normalized to the maximum force evoked at the beginning of fatigue testing (t = 0 sec) by the specific muscle.

The stimulation amplitude required to evoke a forceful contraction depended on electrode placement. In all cases, lower voltages were found with the cathodic lead located in close proximity to the main nerve bundles. Intramuscular electrodes (impedance = 400 ohm) required stimulation amplitudes of 3 to 5 V, depending on electrode position. Impedance and threshold pulse amplitudes remained stable with time. No mechanical and electrochemical problems with Pt/Ir electrodes were encountered.

Electrophysiological measurements showed that conditioned muscles were slower than their contralaterals (Fig. 2). Burst stimulation at increasing frequencies demonstrated that the fusion frequency was consequently lower for conditioned muscles. Fusion was investigated by measuring the relative force ripple at different burst frequencies (Fig. 3). A fused contraction was defined as one having a peak-to-peak ripple less than 2% of the peak force. Burst-conditioned muscles exhibited the lowest fusion frequency (12 $\pm$ 3 Hz). Fusion

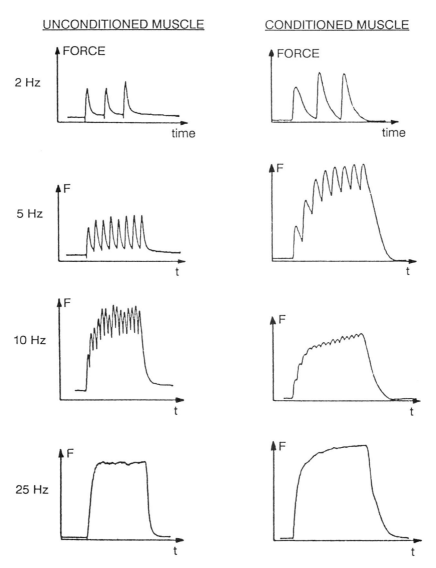

Figure 2. *Electrophysiological studies. LDM tetanization obtained with increased stimulation frequency for conditioned and unconditioned muscles.*

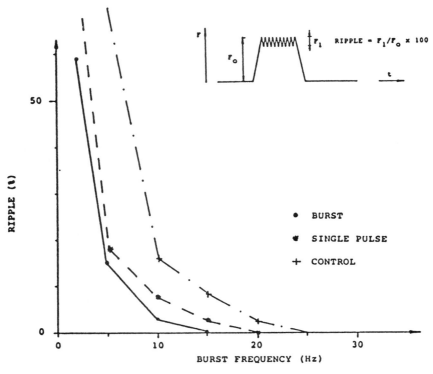

Figure 3. *Ripple variation with burst frequency.*

frequencies were 16 ± 5 Hz for single pulse conditioning and 24 ± 4 Hz for contralateral controls (Table 2).

The fatigue resistance characteristics were estimated by measuring the relative evoked force decrease after 15 minutes of cyclic stimulation (Fig. 4). Force decrease was lower for the conditioned muscles ($-22\% \pm 4\%$, single pulse; $-20\% \pm 4\%$, burst) than for their contralateral unconditioned muscle ($-50\% \pm 6\%$) (Table 2).

Table 2
Comparative Electrophysiological Results

	Unconditioned	Conditioned	
		Single Pulse	Burst
Fusion Frequency (Hz)	24 ± 4 Hz	16 ± 5 Hz	12 ± 3 Hz
Fatigue Resistance (force decrease after 15 min exercise)	$-50\% \pm 6\%$	$-22\% \pm 4\%$	$-20\% \pm 4\%$

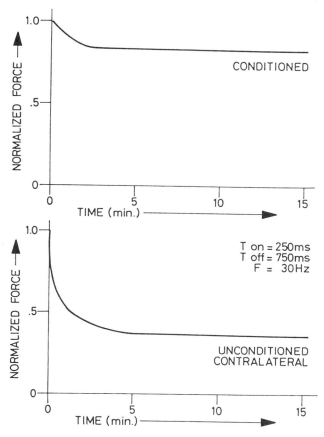

Figure 4. *Muscle fatigue test. Force decreases after 15 minutes of exercise shows a significant difference between conditioned and unconditioned muscle.*

Histochemical Study

Biopsies of the proximal and distal portions of the conditioned latissimus dorsi muscle were performed. A biopsy of the contralateral unconditioned latissimus dorsi was also taken for comparison. The goal of this histochemical and histopathological study was to evaluate muscle conversion (fast glycolitic fatigable fibers into slow oxidative fatigue-resistant fibers) as well as to determine occasional myofibrillar alterations after long-term sequential electrical stimulation.

Histochemical studies showed significant differences among the various groups of animals (Fig. 5). In the group of muscles stimulated with a "pulse-train protocol" (bursts), the percentage of slow-twitch fatigue-resistant fibers was greater than in muscles stimulated with the "single pulse protocol" and the later greater than in the "unconditioned control muscles" (Table 3). The histologic muscle structure was always retained, and no degenerative or inflammatory reaction was seen (Fig. 6).

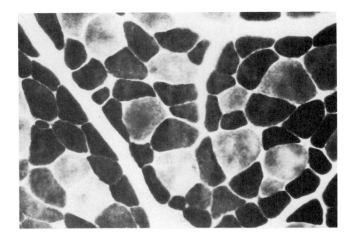

Figure 5A. *Histochemical study of nonstimulated control LDM. (Cross section stained for myofibrillar ATPase [pH 9.4]). Light-stained fibers are classified as type I, slow-twitch oxidative, fatigue-resistant fibers. Dark-stained fibers as type II, fast-twitch, gly-colytic fatigue-prone fibers.*

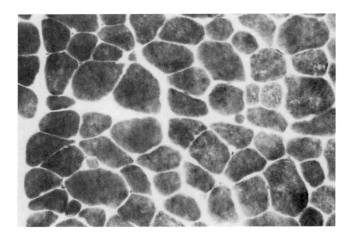

Figure 5B. *LDM stimulated by pulse trains (30 Hz) for 6 months. Complete conversion to type I, oxidative fibers.*

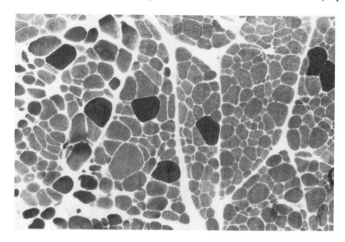

Figure 5C. *LDM stimulated by single pulses for two years. Incomplete conversion.*

In this experience we showed that burst conditioning with a 6–month follow-up provided a better fiber conversion than single pulse training with a 2-year follow-up. The slight differences found in fusion frequency and fatigue resistance between these two groups is probably due to the different conditioning period duration.

Effect of Cardiomyoplasty on Ventricular Function

Method

The effect of cardiomyoplasty on ventricular function was studied in an experiment on 10 adult female goats weighing 47–59 kg and followed for up to 9 months.[11] The left latissimus dorsi muscle flap was dissected, while keeping the axillary pedicle intact. Two intramuscular electrodes (Medtronic Model

Table 3 Histochemical Results		
	% Slow-Twitch Oxidative Fibers (acid stain)	*% Slow-Twitch Oxidative Fibers (alkaline stain)*
Conditioned Muscles (Pulse Trains, 6 months)	99% ± 1%	94% ± 5%
Conditioned Muscles (Single Pulses, 2 years)	87% ± 7%	83% ± 8%
Unconditioned Muscles	46% ± 5%	42% ± 7%

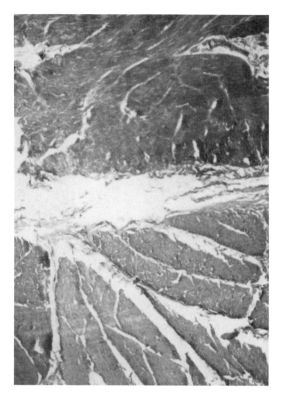

Figure 6. *Muscle-myocardium interface 6 months postoperatively shows no histological alteration of muscle or myocardium.*

SP5528), designed by Chachques and manufactured for high fatigue resistance, were implanted in the upper part of the latissimus dorsi muscle flap (pedicle area). The proximal electrode (cathode) was placed near the motor nerve branches, slightly distal to their penetration into the muscle. The distal electrode was placed 6–8 cm more distally (Fig. 7). Controlled electrophysiological isotonic measurements were performed on the latissimus dorsi muscle flap, stimulated by an external pulse generator. In order to evaluate the degree of shortening of the muscle and the force developed during stimulation, the anterior limb was immobilized and weights of 200–1,000 g were connected to the most distal part of the muscle with a system of pulleys (Fig. 8). A brief maximum stimulation was achieved with the following characteristics: 30–Hz, 185-ms burst duration and 30 contractions/min. Isotonic muscular contractions showed that during muscle stimulation the muscle shortening relative to the muscle maximum physiological length decreased as the load increased from 46% with a 200-g load to 19% at a 1000-g load (Fig. 9).

The muscle flap and the leads then were transferred into the thoracic cavity by way of a partial (5 cm) resection of the anterior part of the second rib. Thoracotomy at the fifth left intercostal space and pericardiotomy were

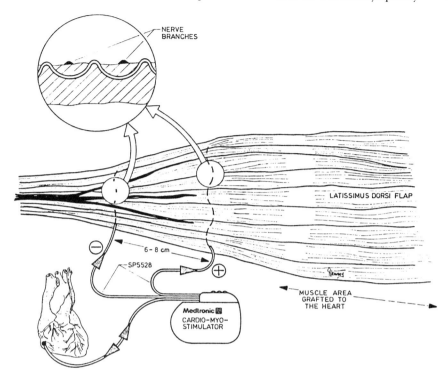

Figure 7. *Placement of skeletal muscle pacing electrodes (Medtronic Model SP5528). The cathodic lead (−) located near the nerve branches results in strong contraction of the entire latissimus dorsi muscle.*

used to expose the heart. A sensing electrode (Medtronic Model SP5548) was implanted in the right ventricular wall and was subsequently used to detect the ventricular signal. The latissimus dorsi muscle flap then was wrapped around both ventricles and fixed with interrupted sutures. Electrodes were coupled to a Cardiomyostimulator™ Pulse Train Generator (Medtronic Model SP1005) equipped with a sensing chamber and a pacing chamber to deliver either single pulses or bursts of pulses for chronic muscle stimulation in synchrony with the cardiac rhythm. Muscle stimulation parameters were the following: synchronization delay 4 ms, pulse amplitude 4–5 V, pulse width 210 μs, burst rate 30 Hz, and burst duration 185 ms. The amplitude of the R wave was recorded during implantation of the cardiac lead and monitored during the entire follow-up period. Two implantable ultrasonic probes (5 MHz), fixed on the aorta and on the pulmonary artery in four goats, were coupled postoperatively to an ultrasonic Doppler instrument (Vingmed SD 100, Vingmed, Horten, Norway) to provide quantitative hemodynamic information. The other six animals were studied with ultrasonic external transducers.

The protocol of progressive sequential stimulation of the skeletal muscle,[9] coordinated with the systolic-diastolic cycle, started with a single impulse

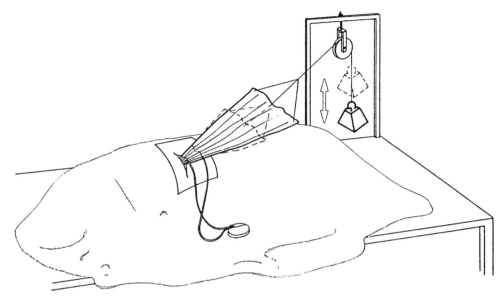

Figure 8. *Latissimus dorsi electrophysiological study. Method for measurement of iso-tonic muscular contractions.*

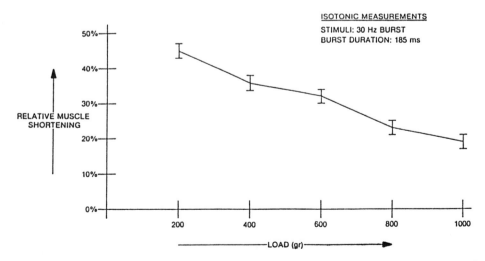

Figure 9. *Relative LDMF shortening (%) versus load (gr) during burst-impulse muscle stimulation (n = 10).*

followed by bursts of impulses (synchronization delay 4 ms). As shown above, a single-pulse stimulation results in a single-twitch evoked force (Fig. 2). Larger and longer muscular contraction can be obtained by multiple stimulation pulses (burst of impulses) spaced in time in such a way that temporal summation occurs. The duration of contraction duration can be physiologically adapted to ventricular systolic activity. In our muscle-stimulation protocol (experimental and clinical), we used bursts of impulses composed of 210 µs balanced cathodic pulses occurring at a frequency of 30 Hz. This stimulation rate (30 Hz) generates action potentials occurring at frequencies similar to those of natural physiological nerve discharges. A duty cycle of chronic muscle electrostimulation, with the stimulation on 25% of the time (185 ms burst duration) and off 75% of the time (555 ms) (synchronization ratio 1:1, 81 pulses/min), has been shown to produce repeated and sustained muscle work without significant fatigue, fiber degeneration, or both.

Electrostimulation began 2 weeks after cardiomyoplasty (Fig. 10). The latissimus dorsi muscle flap was progressively put into use by slowly increasing the burst frequency content, that is, number of pulses as well as the heart-muscle contraction ratio (2:1, 1:1). After 2 months, all animals were stimulated with pulse trains. The intramuscular electrode length within the latissimus dorsi muscle was 40 ± 5 mm at the proximal pedicle site (cathode) and 100 ± 10 mm at the distal site (anode). The interelectrode distance was 70 ± 10 mm. At the time of implantation, the stimulation threshold (measured at a 0.2 ms pulse width) was 0.8 ± 0.3 V and the lead impedance was 350 ± 50

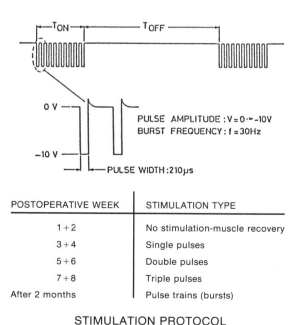

POSTOPERATIVE WEEK	STIMULATION TYPE
1 + 2	No stimulation-muscle recovery
3 + 4	Single pulses
5 + 6	Double pulses
7 + 8	Triple pulses
After 2 months	Pulse trains (bursts)

STIMULATION PROTOCOL

Figure 10. *Latissimus dorsi electrostimulation protocol following cardiomyoplasty.*

ohm. At the postoperative follow-up assessment, the stimulation threshold increased to 1.0 ± 0.3 V and the impedance increased to 380 ± 80 ohm. In all cases, a forceful contraction could be evoked with bursts of impulses of amplitude 3.5 ± 0.5 V. R-wave amplitude was 13 ± 5 mV at the time of implantation. This signal was always adequate to properly synchronize the Cardiomyostimulator™ Pulse Train Generator.

This protocol of progressive sequential stimulation takes into account not only the delay of the gradual conversion of fast-twitch glycolytic fatigue-prone muscular fibers to slow-twitch oxydative fatigue-resistant fibers but also the healing time required by the muscle to recover collateral blood circulation and to adhere to the heart. The adhesion between the external surface of the latissimus dorsi muscle flap and the pericardium is also important to avoid upper traction of the heart during muscle stimulation and its hemodynamic consequences.

Ventricular Function

Nine months after cardiomyoplasty, the cardiac output was measured by a thermodilution technique with a cardiac output computer (American Edwards Model 9520, Irvine, California) coupled to a Swan-Ganz catheter with the Cardiomyostimulator™ Pulse Train Generator in the "ON" and "OFF" position (10 minutes).[11] A significant increase in cardiac output was detected in all animals during burst electrical stimulation of the muscle flap, from 3.81 ± 0.16 L/min (with the Cardiomyostimulator™ Pulse Train Generator "OFF") to 4.57 ± 0.19 L/min (with the Cardiomyostimulator™ Pulse Train Generator "ON") (p < 0.025). Hemodynamic studies were further conducted by inducing myocardial failure using high dose of propranolol (3 mg/kg intravenously). A significant increase in left ventriuclar pressures was obtained after stimulation Fig. 11. Ultrasonic Doppler measurements showed that synchronous burst

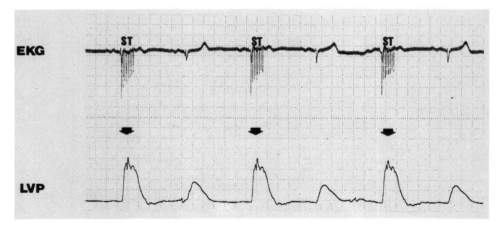

Figure 11. *Hemodynamic study following reinforcement cardiomyoplasty. Temporary myocardial failure was induced in goats, using high doses of propranolol (3 mg/ kg/ intravenously). Increase of left ventricular pressure (LVP) during LDMF stimulation (ST). Heart:muscle stimulation ratio 2.1.*

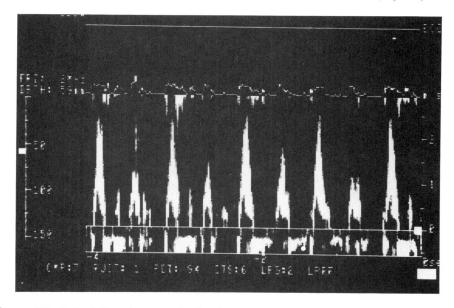

Figure 12. *Pulsed-Doppler record of pulmonary artery systolic flow after cardiomyoplasty. Muscle flap stimulation 2.1. Increase in blood velocity is demonstrated during stimulated cycles.*

stimulation of the muscle flap increased the blood peak velocity in the descending aorta ($+40\% \pm 6\%$) and increased the left ventricular stroke volume ($+98\% \pm 10\%$). Measurement of the pulmonary artery flow showed an $81\% \pm 9\%$ increase in blood peak velocity (Fig. 12), while the right ventricular stroke volume increased by $102\% \pm 14\%$ (Table 4). After the hemodynamic

Table 4
Ultrasonic Doppler Measurements After
Cardiomyoplasty

Parameter	Measurement
Ventricular Stroke Volume	
Left ventricle	$+$ 98% $+/-$ 10%
Right ventricle	$+$ 102% $+/-$ 14%
Blood Peak Velocity	
Aorta	$+$ 40% $+/-$ 6%
Pulmonary artery	$+$ 81% $+/-$ 9%

Values shown are relative increase of ventricular stroke volume and blood peak velocity due to synchronous electrical stimulation (30-Hz bursts) of the muscle flap from the follow-up assessment at 9 months (n = 10).

investigations were completed, the animals were put to death in order to perform histological, histochemical, and biochemical studies.

Histology

Histological studies showed essentially no fibrosis, fiber atrophy, or degeneration in any part of the muscle flaps, including the areas of electrode implantation. Encapsulation surrounding the electrodes pairs was always thin (<0.5 mm), and the muscular cytoarchitecture surrounding the electrodes at the cathodic and anodic sites was intact. Electron microscopy showed preserved myofibrillar structure, increased capillary density, and increased mitochondrial cell volume. It was possible to see a few collagen fibers between the myocardial surface and the skeletal muscle with small anastomotic vessels. No evidence of inflammatory or degenerative reaction was seen.

Histochemistry and Biochemistry

Histochemical studies showed that in stimulated latissimus dorsi muscle flaps, the percentage of slow-twitch oxidative fatigue-resistant fibers was greater than that in contralateral control muscles (99% ± 1% vs 31% ± 3%) (Fig. 13). The histochemical muscle characteristics were always retained and no evidence of degenerative reaction was seen. The mean diameter of oxidative

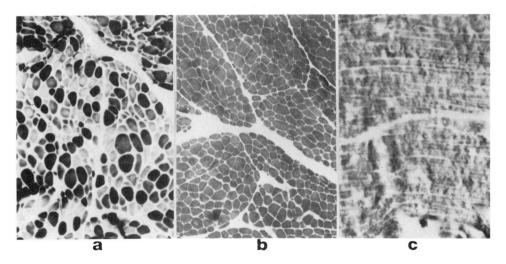

Figure 13. *Photomicrographs documenting histochemical studies of LDM fibers and myocardium. ATPase staining, ×322. a. Nonstimulated control muscle. b. LDM electrostimulated by pulse trains for 9 months showing the complete conversion from type II glycolytic to type I oxidative fibers. c. Control myocardium shows similar histochemical characteristics as stimulated LDM.*

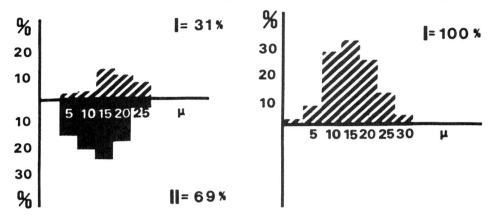

Figure 14. *A (left). Histogram of control nonstimulated LDM: distribution of oxidative (I) and glycolytic (II) fibers, and fiber diameter measurement (μ). B (right). After 9 months of LDM electrostimulation, there is complete histochemical transformation to oxidative type fibers with similar fiber diameters.*

electrostimulated fibers was 17 ± 2.5 μ. In control muscles, the mean diameter of fibers was 17 ± 3 μ (oxidative) and 14 ± 2 μ (glycolytic) (Fig. 14).

Electrophoretic analysis was carried out with two types of electrophoresis (native gel and SDS-PAGE) to separate fast and slow myosin isoforms. These two methods yield complementary results: native gel analysis resolves the entire myosin molecule, whereas SDS-PAGE analysis specifically resolves the heavy chains. Native gels typical of myosins in contralateral and stimulated latissimus dorsi muscles are shown in Figure 15 together with rat extensorum digitorum longus and rat soleus. In the control (Fig. 15, lane 1), the predom-

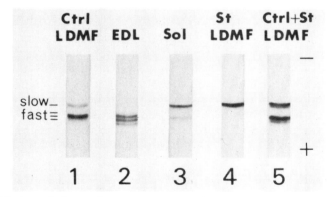

Figure 15. *Native gel electrophoresis of myosins from control (Ctrl) and stimulated (St) LDMF. Migration was from (−) to (+): lane 1, control LDM; lane 2, control rat extensorum digitorum longus (EDL); lane 3, control rat soleus (Sol); lane 4, stimulated LDMF; and lane 5, control + stimulated LDMF. Approximately 2 μg myosin was loaded in each gel.*

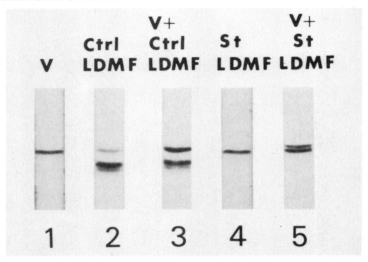

Figure 16. *Native gel electrophoresis of myosins from control (Ctrl) and stimulated (St) LDMF and from ventricular (V) tissue. Migration was from − to +; lane 1, ventricle; lane 2, control LDM; lane 3, ventricle + control LDM; lane 4, stimulated LDMF; and lane 5, stimulated LDMF + ventricle.*

inant forms are the fast isoforms that migrate approximately at the same velocity as those from rat muscles (Fig. 15, lane 2) with a small amount of slow isomyosin whose migration is similar to that of rat soleus (Fig. 15, lane 3). In stimulated latissimus dorsi muscle flaps (Fig. 15, lane 4), the slow isoform was the only one present, and the fast isoforms had completely disappeared. Comigration of myosins from contralateral and stimulated muscles nevertheless indicated that the slow myosin from stimulated muscle was not completely identical to that of the contralateral control muscle (see doublet on Fig. 15, lane 5).

In all animal species tested so far, the slow isomyosin of ventricular tissue is the same as that of slow-twitch muscle fibers. In Figure 16, the native gel electrophoresis pattern of goat ventricular myosin is compared with that of control and stimulated latissimus dorsi muscles. Goat ventricular myosin (Fig. 16, lane 1) has exactly the same electrophoretic mobility as the slow isoform of the contralateral control latissimus dorsi muscle (Fig. 16, lane 2), and indeed, comigrations indicated only one band (lane 3). However, comigration of myosins from stimulated latissimus dorsi muscle flaps and ventricular tissue again evidenced two bands (Fig. 16, lane 5), confirming that the myosin from stimulated latissimus dorsi muscle flap was slightly different from that of slow cardiac muscle.

To determine whether the differences were attributable to the heavy chains, analysis of slow myosin heavy chains was accomplished by electrophoresis under denaturing conditions in the presence of low-percentage polyacrylamide gel that allows a good separation between fast and slow myosin heavy chains. Figure 17 shows that slow myosin heavy chains from the stimulated latissimus dorsi muscle flap (Fig. 17, lane 1) yield an electrophoretic

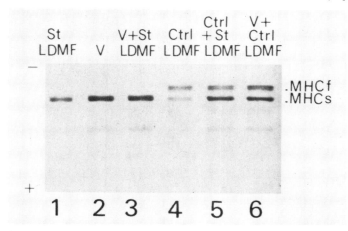

Figure 17. *Sodium dodecyl sulfate polyacrylamide gel electrophoresis (SDS-PAGE) of myosin heavy chain fast (MHCf) and slow (MHCs) isoforms of LDMF and ventricular (V) tissue. About 100 μg of protein per lane: lane 1, stimulated (St) LDMF; lane 2, ventricle (V); lane 3, stimulated LDMF + ventricle; lane 4, control LDM; lane 5, control LDM + stimulated LDMF; lane 6, control LDM + ventricle. Note that all MHCs yield one band, even in the comigration experiments.*

pattern identical to that of ventricular tissue (Fig. 17, lane 2), even in comigration experiments (Fig. 17, lane 3). In latissimus dorsi control muscles (Fig. 17, lane 4), fast and slow myosin heavy chains were present, which correlates well with the results obtained by native gel electrophoresis. Comigration of control and stimulated latissimus dorsi muscle (Fig. 17, lane 5) and of control latissimus dorsi muscle and ventricular tissue (Fig. 17, lane 6) resolved only one band at the level of slow myosin heavy chains. Taken all together, these results indicate that stimulation of latissimus dorsi muscle flaps induces the complete replacement of fast myosin heavy chain by its slow counterpart. The difference that is evidenced by native gel electrophoresis most likely is due to an incomplete transformation of the light chains.

Changes in the myosin light and heavy chain complement from electrical stimulation were first reported by Salmons,[12] and his findings subsequently have been confirmed and extended.[13,14] Replacement of the fast by the slow isoforms of individual light and heavy chains of native myosin does not occur synchronously as the heavy chains are replaced before the light chains. Indeed, we found complete replacement of the fast by the slow cardiac type of myosin heavy chain (Fig. 17), whereas it is probable that the light chains are not completely transformed. One might hypothesize that, with more prolonged stimulation, the fast light chains would also completely disappear. Replacement of the fast by the slow cardiac type heavy chains would be expected to result in a significant reduction of the velocity of the muscle shortening since the velocity of shortening in fibers composed of both myosin types is highly correlated with the myosin heavy chain composition with velocity increasing as the proportion of fast heavy chains increases. This did not seem to compromise the effect of cardiomyoplasty on ventricular function in our experiments since velocity remained within the range required for adequate assistance.

References

1. Leriche R, Fontaine R: Essai, expérimental de traitement de certains infarctus du myocarde et de l'anévrysme du coeur par une greffe de muscle strié. Bull Soc Nat Chir 59:229, 1933.
2. Petrovsky BV: Surgical treatment of cardiac aneurysms. J Cardiovasc Surg 7:87, 1966.
3. Christ J, Spira M: Application of the latissimus dorsi muscle to the heart. Ann Plast Surg 8:118, 1982.
4. Kantrowitz A, McKinnon WMP: The experimental use of the diaphragm as an auxiliary myocardium. Surg Forum 9:266, 1959.
5. Termet H, Chalencon JL, Estour E, et al: Transplantation sur le myocarde d'un muscle strié excité par pacemaker. Ann Chir Thorac Cardiovasc 5:568, 1966.
6. Macoviak JA, Stephenson LW, Spielman S: Replacement of ventricular myocardium with diapraghmatic skeletal muscles. J Thorac Cardiovasc Surg 81:519, 1981.
7. Chachques JC, Mitz V, Hero M, et al: Transfert d'un muscle innervé sur le coeur. In G Magalon, V Mitz (eds): Les Lambeaux pédiculés musculaires et musculo-cutanés. Paris, Masson, 1984, pp 5–6.
8. Dewar HL, Drinkwater DC, Chiu RC-J: Synchronously stimulated skeletal muscle graft for myocardial repair: an experimental study. J Thorac Cardiovasc Surg 87:325, 1987.
9. Carpentier A, Chachques JC, Grandjean PA, et al: Transformation d'un muscle squelettique par stimulation séquentielle progressive en vue de son utilisation comme substitut myocardique. CR Acad Sci Paris 301:581, 1985.
10. Chachques JC, Grandjean PA, Carpentier A: Dynamic cardiomyoplasty: experimental cardiac wall replacement with a stimulated skeletal muscle. In RC-J Chiu (ed): Biomechanical Cardiac Assist: Cardiomyoplasty and Muscle-Powered Devices. Mount Kisco, NY, Futura Publishing Co, 1986, pp 59–84.
11. Chachques JC, Grandjean P, Schwartz K, et al: Effect of latissimus dorsi dynamic cardiomyoplasty on ventricular function. Circulation 78(Suppl 3):203, 1988.
12. Salmons S, Henriksson J: The adaptative response of skeletal muscle to increase use. Muscle Nerve 4:94, 1981.
13. Adams RJ, Schwartz A: comparative mechanisms for contraction of cardiac and skeletal muscle. Chest 78:123, 1980.
14. Brown WE, Salmons S, Whalen RG: The sequential replacement of myosin subunit isoforms during muscle type transformation induced by long term electrical stimulation. J Biol Chem 258:14686, 1983.

Part II
Surgical Technique and Clinical Experience

Chapter 7

Preoperative Management and Anesthesia

Danielle Bensasson, Jean Philippe Kieffer

The first cardiomyoplasty was performed by Carpentier and his team in January 1985.[1,2] Since then 19 additional cases have been carried out in the same institution and significant improvements have been made in the preoperative and intraoperative management of those high-risk patients. The desperate condition of these patients preoperatively, the lengthy operation, and the operative lateral decubitus position with its subsequent disorder in lung ventilation and perfusion caused specific problems for the anesthesiologist that are analyzed in this chapter.

Preoperative Conditions and Management

Among 20 patients operated on between January 1985 and June 1989, 10 were in functional Class IV (NYHA) and 10 in functional Class III. Six patients required either intra-aortic balloon counterpulsation or biventricular assist prior to or during surgery. Seven patients displayed ventricular extrasystoles. Two of these patients had experienced several brief episodes of ventricular tachycardia. Eight patients had renal failure, 7 had diabetes, 14 were heavy smokers, and 3 had chronic obstructive pulmonary disease (CPOD). Ejection fraction, excluding ventricular aneurysm whenever present, ranged from 9% to 27% (mean 15.4%).

The preparation of anesthesia was found to be of primary importance because of the poor condition of the patients selected. The patients with CPOD were all submitted to a 3-week preoperative pulmonary preparation including postural drainage, antibiotherapy, and deep breathing and coughing exercises. The numerous drugs taken by the patient, including calcium channel blockers, diuretics, antiarrhythmics, nitrates, and angiotensin-converting enzyme inhibitors, were administered up to the day before surgery and prescribed thereafter.

From *Cardiomyoplasty* edited by Alain Carpentier, MD, PhD, Juan-Carlos Chachques, MD, and Pierre Grandjean, MS © 1991. Futura Publishing Inc., Mount Kisco, NY.

Anesthesia

Since induction carries a special risk in this group of patients of a potential arterial pressure drop, inotropic drugs (dobutamine 5 µg/kg/min) and intra-aortic balloon counterpulsation were instituted systematically when systolic blood pressure was <90 mm Hg.

Anesthesia was administered using phenoperidine (50 µg/kg), flunitrazepam (30 µg/kg) and thiopental (3 mg/kg). A nasotracheal tube was introduced after neuromuscular blockade by atracurium (500 µg/kg) and local anesthesia of the glottis. Anesthesia was maintained with intermittent boluses of phenoperidine and flunitrazepam. Atracurium was prefered because of its short-term action (35 min). One additional bolus of atracurium was given before the patient was placed in the lateral decubitus position. No additional bolus was given until the muscle stimulation thresholds were tested.

The lateral decubitus position used during the first stage of the operation required particular attention since in this position gravity causes a vertical gradient in the distribution of pulmonary flow. The upper lung is well ventilated but poorly perfused and the lower lung well perfused but poorly ventilated resulting in a mismatching of ventilation and perfusion (Fig. 1). A servo ventilator with 5 to 10 mm Hg PEEP was used to improve the ventilation of the lower lung during the procedure except when the muscle flap was transferred into the thorax and during the wrapping of the heart where manual ventilation was necessary to reduce the risk of hypoventilation and arrhythmia. In an unstable cardiac condition, this situation can be the source of serious complications. In one of our patients, the PaO_2, which was 186 mm Hg in the dorsal decubitus position, dropped to 56 mm Hg in the lateral decubitus position. This severe hypoxia did not respond to positive end-expiratory pressure nor to manual ventilation and we decided not to perform the operation.

The introduction of the muscle flap into the chest may further impair pulmonary function. PaO_2 measured at the beginning of the operation with

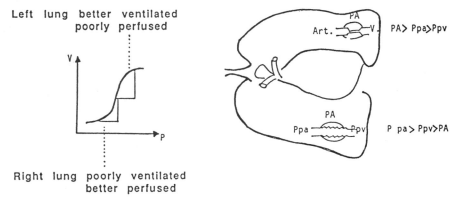

Figure 1. *Pulmonary flow distribution and ventilation in patients in the lateral decubitus position. PA = alveolar pressure.*

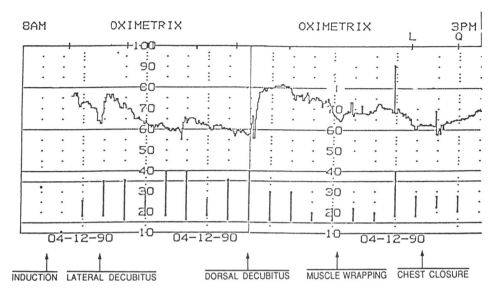

Figure 2. *SVO₂ allows careful monitoring of the patient at the different steps of the operation.*

the patient still in the dorsal decubitus position and then during the latissimus dorsi dissection and transfer into the chest with the patient in the lateral decubitus position showed no significant change in 11 cases and a decrease of more than 50% in 8 cases. This was managed by manual ventilation with a 100 FiO_2 rather than PEEP. Despite this procedure, three patients remained hypoxic. The continuous measurement of SVO_2 was particularly important in the management of these patients (Fig. 2).

Beside ventilatory assistance, all patients required some sort of circulatory support (Table 1). Six patients required dobutamine (4 to 12 μg/kg/mn) during

Table 1
Patient Condition and Cardiac Vascular Support

Severe Cardiac Dysfunction (13 patients, 61%)	
Induction	4
Lateral decubitus	3
During cardiomyoplasty	6
Inotropic Support (15 patients, 75.1%)	
Dobutamine (4 to 15 μg/kg/mn)	11
Isoprenaline (0.04 to 0.1 μg/kg/mn)	4
Epinephrine (0.05 to 0.1 μg/kg/mn)	4
Circulatory Support (5 Patients, 25%)	
I.A.B.C.P.	5
Pierce assistance	1

the induction period. Nitroglycerin (1 μg/kg/mn) was given at the beginning of the operation in 18 of 20 cases. Half of the patients received dopamine (3 μg/kg/min) during the entire procedure because of preoperative renal failure. The diabetic patients, whether insulin-dependent or not were treated by continuous intravenous insulin during the procedure to maintain the glycemia around 8 mmol/L.

Complications

Low Cardiac Output

In spite of all precautions taken, 12 patients presented a low cardiac output. This was treated successfully by inotropic drugs in 6 patients and 6 patients required circulatory assistance. Of the 6 patients requiring circulatory assistance, aortic counterpulsation was used in 5 patients and left and right support with Pierce Thoratec ventricles in 1 patient.

Severe Arrhythmias

All patients presented some kind of arrhythmia at some time during the operation (Table 2). Ectopic beats were the most commonly encountered anomaly. Severe ventricular arrhythmias usually were associated with hypoxemia. In one case irreversible ventricular fibrillation led to patient death in the operating room. A prophylaxis using systematic lidocaine may be advisable.

Table 2 Incidence of Arrhythmia During Operation	
Ventricular fibrillation	3
Ventricular tachycardia	2
Atrial fibrillation	3
AV block	1
Premature ventricular contractions	15

Risk Factors

The exact factors influencing the outcome of this procedure are difficult to establish because of the small number of patients. However, some common preoperative findings were encountered in most patients who presented intraoperative complications and ultimately died (Table 3). From our early experience with two patients who did not survive the operation, we have learned that a cardiac index less than 1.3 L/mn/m² and/or a CWP over 40 mm Hg or

Table 3
Risk Factors and Death

	Patients	Deaths
Functional Class IV	15	6
Severe arrhythmia preop.	4	2
CWP > 30	8	3
Renal failure	7	5
Recent pulmonary edema	8	5
Valvular lesions	3	3

LVEDP > 50 mm Hg with signs of right heart failure, ascitis, and edema should be considered as contraindications to the procedure.

References

1. Carpentier A, Chachques JC, Grandjean PA: Transformation d'un muscle squelettique par stimulation sequentielle progressive en vue de son utilisation comme substitut myocardique. CR Acad Sc Paris 301:581, 1985.
2. Carpentier A, Chachques JC: Myocardial substitution with a stimulated skeletal muscle: first successful clinical case. Lancet 1:1267, 1985.

Chapter 8

Cardiomyoplasty: Surgical Technique

Alain Carpentier, Juan-Carlos Chachques*

Since the first clinical case of cardiomyoplasty in 1965,[1,2] the surgical technique has undergone several changes in an attempt to increase the efficiency of the operation and to decrease the operative risk.[3,4] These changes concern the timing of muscle stimulation, the surgical approach to the heart, the use of extracorporeal circulation, the orientation of the muscle flap, and the technique of fixation of the muscle to the heart. This chapter concentrates on the technique currently in use, which is the result of these changes.

It must be understood that cardiomyoplasty is not an ordinary surgical operation, carried out on ordinary surgical patients. The procedure consists of two steps: latissimus dorsi mobilization and wrapping of the heart. The patients are in the final stage of heart failure. They have fragile and excitable ventricles that are inclined to fibrillate and difficult to defibrillate. Under these circumstances, all surgical details are of extreme importance.

Latissimus Dorsi Mobilization

The left latissimus dorsi is the muscle of choice because of its large muscular mass and its ability to be transferred into the thorax while preserving its neurovascular pedicle.[5] The mobilization of the muscle and the cardiomyoplasty itself are carried out during the same operation. In the beginning of our experience, however, a two-stage operation was attempted with the hope that a preconditioned muscle could be used immediately after the operation. This was not possible however as a 2-week period of nonstimulation proved to be necessary to facilitate adhesion between the heart and the muscle. At the end of that period, the muscle had lost most of its fatigue-resistant characteristics requiring another similar period of progressive sequential stimulation.

The following is a description of the one-stage technique recommended

* With the cooperation of P Perier and C Acar.
From *Cardiomyoplasty* edited by Alain Carpentier, MD, PhD, Juan-Carlos Chachques, MD, and Pierre Grandjean, MS © 1991. Futura Publishing Inc., Mount Kisco, NY.

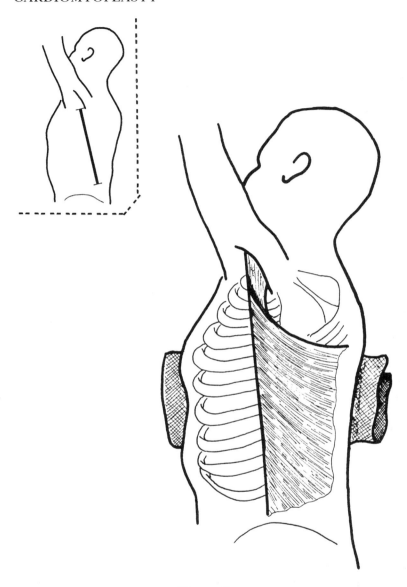

Figure 1.

today. The patient is placed in a right lateral decubitus position with the left arm elevated (Fig. 1). The muscle is approached through a vertical skin incision extending from the posterior edge of the axillary region to the midpoint of the twelfth rib. Once the subcutaneous tissues have been incised, the edges of the skin incision are covered by drapes sutured to the subcutaneous tissues so as to avoid any contact of the muscle with the skin and therefore to minimize the risk of infection. The latissimus dorsi is dissected free from all insertions.

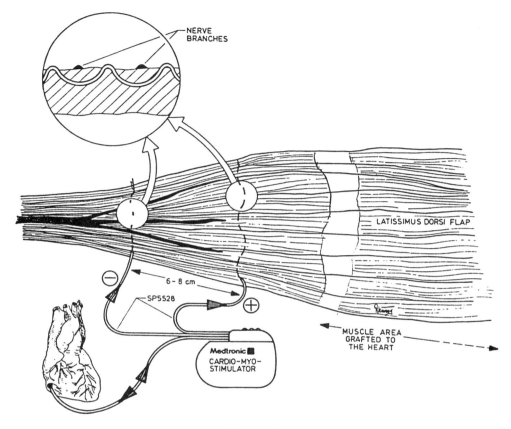

Figure 2.

Its humeral tendon is cut with theexception of its posterior fascia so as to carefully preserve the thoracodorsal neurovascular pedicle. Electrodes specially designed for long term muscle stimulation (Medtronic Model SP5528) are implanted. Both electrodes are made of a platinum iridium alloy and have a 5-cm stimulating wire that provides a large area of contact with the muscular fibers. The negative lead is located at the point of penetration of the nerve branches into the muscle and the positive lead is located 6 to 8 cm more distally (Fig. 2). The electrodes are passed superficially within the muscle so as not to compromise the nerve and the vascular branches. An external pulse generator is used temporarily to measure the thresholds and the efficacy of the stimulation. Stimulation *threshold* must be inferior to 3V.

A window is then created into the chest by removing the anterior third (5 cm) of the second rib. Through this window, the muscle flap is transferred into the thorax together with the electrodes (Fig. 3). The proximal part of the muscle is sutured to the periosteum of the third rib so as to prevent any traction on the vascular pedicle. After careful hemostasis and placement of several drainage tubes in the area of dissection, the subcutaneous tissues and the skin

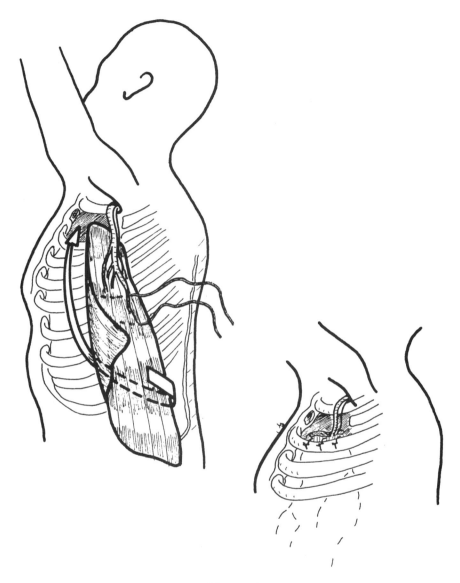

Figure 3.

are sutured carefully. Since seroma formation underneath the skin flaps is common, it is important to suture the subcutaneous tissue in multiple places to the chest wall.

Cardiomyoplasty

The technique of cardiomyoplasty has evolved throughout the years. The first difficult decision was whether the heart should be approached through a

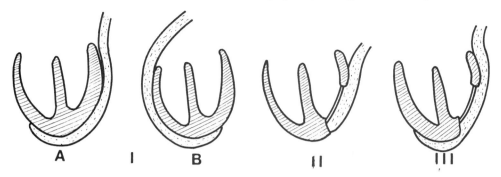

Figure 4.

left thoracotomy taking advantage of the lateral decubitus position necessary for the latissimus dorsi mobilization or through a median sternotomy, which provides better access to the heart and does not impair lung function. We have used the left thoracotomy approach only once and have subsequently found the median sternotomy more appropriate since associated procedures on the ventricles, the valves, or coronary arteries are often necessary. Another advantage of the two-incision technique is that it separates the chest cavity from the area of latissimus dorsi mobilization, which is a potential site for infection given the large area of dissection. Another difficult decision was whether or not extracorporeal circulation should be used routinely. Initially, we used it in all patients. We now find it preferable to avoid extracorporeal circulation whenever possible. This policy has reduced the amount of bleeding in the area of latissimus dorsi dissection and the risk of infection. In addition, it seems to facilitate a more rapid postoperative recovery of the patient. Special attention has been given to the fixation of the muscle to the heart. Several techniques were tried to minimize heart mobilization and injury to the myocardium. The development in 1988 of the "no myocardial suture technique" was particularly important in this regard and is still our technique of choice.

There are three cardiomyoplasty techniques the choice of which depends on the lesions encountered:

· The "reinforcement technique" or muscular wrapping of the ventricles (used in 13 cases in our experience).
· The "substitution technique" or muscular patching of a myocardial defect after resection of a large aneurysm or a tumor (used in 2 cases).
· The combined "substitution and reinforcement technique" in patients with a large aneurysm and poor function of the remaining ventricle (5 cases) (Fig. 4).

The Reinforcement Technique

The reinforcement technique can be carried out using one of two different modalities: anterior wrapping or posterior wrapping, depending on the size of the heart, the length of the muscle, and which ventricle is the most affected by the underlying disease.

Posterior Wrapping

Posterior wrapping is the most frequently used modality because the heart is generally big and the muscle is too short to cover the two ventricles. In addition the left ventricle being the most affected must be wrapped first. Posterior wrapping has been used in 12 cases in our experience.

After the left latissimus dorsi has been dissected and transferred into the thorax, the patient is placed in a supine position. The extracorporeal circulation circuit is prepared and filled with the priming solution. A median sternotomy is performed, and the chest is open asymmetrically with a predominant opening of the left side to facilitate the exposure and mobilization of the heart (Fig. 5). The left pleural cavity is opened wide enough to expose the anterior aspect of the pericardial sac. The pericardium is incised vertically 0.5 cm from and parallel to the left phrenic nerve (Fig. 5). A pericardial flap attached to the right half of the pericardial sac is tailored by extending the vertical incision transversely at the inferior and superior aspects of the pericardial sac (Fig. 5). The pericardial sac is further incised 2 to 3 cm under the left phrenic nerve to avoid any compression of the latissimus dorsi by a sharp posterior free edge of the pericardial sac.

Pursestring sutures are placed on the aorta and on the right atrium so that rapid cannulation can be accomplished if necessary.

Adhesions whenever present are carefully released. The pericardial sac is thoroughly spread with topical Xylocaine before mobilization is attempted. Because of the versatility of the heart, manipulation must be limited. Several episodes of hypotension during heart manipulation may lead to progressive distension of the ventricles, irreversible damage of the myocardium, and irreversible fibrillation. If mobilization of the heart leads to severe arrhythmias and/or a significant decrease in blood pressure, aortic and venous cannulation is carried out so that, if necessary, extracorporeal circulation can be instituted without delay. The muscle flap is then examined to determine the amount of muscular tissue available and the optimal way it should be wrapped around the heart. The shape of the flap is triangular with two unequal lateral sides and one base. The flap has a subcutaneous (superficial) surface characterized by a smooth regular aspect and a costal (deep) surface characterized by its rough aspect and the penetration of the nerve branches. The longest lateral side of the flap is selected to be placed posterior to the left ventricle. In most instances (16 of 20 cases in our experience), the longest lateral side of the triangle corresponds to the medial edge of the muscle in situ and therefore the subcutaneous surface of the flap is in contact with the epicardium (Fig. 6). In a few instances (4 of 20 cases in our experience), the longest lateral side corresponds to the spinal edge of the in situ muscle and therefore the costal surface of the flap is in contact with the epicardium (Fig. 7).

Once the longest lateral edge of the triangle has been selected, gentle longitudinal traction is applied to the flap and 2–0 resorbable pilot sutures

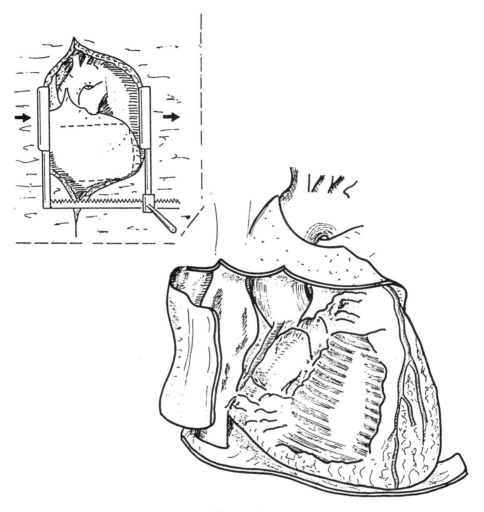

Figure 5.

are placed on this edge. One is placed proximally at the level of the origin of the pulmonary artery trunk, and one is placed distally at the level of the diaphragm near the inferior vena cavae (Fig. 6). These pilot sutures are used to facilitate the positioning of the flap. With the surgeon's left hand, the heart is slightly retracted to the right and upwards . Only a 2- to 3-cm elevation of the apex is needed. With the surgeon's right hand and rightwards gentle traction on pilot sutures, the flap is positioned behind the left ventricle with the longest edge positioned first (Fig. 8). The distal pilot suture is secured to the pericardium in front of the inferior vena cavae and the proximal suture is secured to the remnant of the pericardium below the origin of the left branch of the pulmonary artery (Fig. 9). Care must be taken to insure that the flap

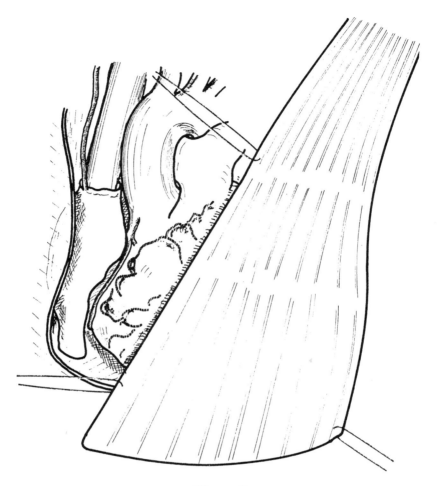

Figure 6.

is not subjected to excess tension nor compressed posteriorly by the pericardium. Two epicardial sensing electrodes (Medtronic Model SP5548) are then placed within the right ventricle — one on the diaphragmatic wall, the other on the anterior wall. A 2- to 3-cm length of the wire must be in contact with myocardium for optimal detection of the QRS complex. The electrodes are tested for proper ventricular signal collection. The minimal acceptable values are a 5 mV amplitude and a 0.5 V/sec slew rate.

The wrapping of the heart is completed by pulling upwards on the base of the flap to cover the diaphragmatic surface of the ventricles and by pulling rightwards on the short lateral side of the triangular flap in order to cover as much of the right ventricle as possible (Fig. 10). These two segments of the muscular flap are then sutured to each other using 4–0 nonresorbable sutures under gentle tension in order to obtain good coaptation between the heart and

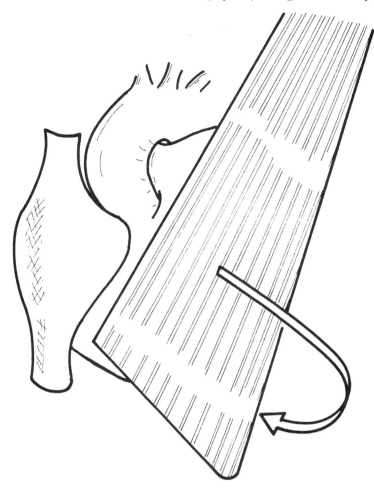

Figure 7.

the flap. Since it is usually not possible to cover the whole anterior aspect of the right ventricle, the pericardial flap tailored at the beginning is used to complete the covering. Its left edge is sutured to the anterior edge of the muscle flap so as to maintain it in proper position (Fig. 11).

At this point, the only part of the two ventricles not covered by the muscle or the pericardial flap is the left border of the heart since it corresponds to the free conoidal space limited by the proximal part of the muscular flap. This free space must be closed so as to cover the left border of the heart. This is achieved by using 4–0 nonresorbable sutures placed superficially between the two layers of the muscular tissue along the left border of the heart.

Three or four additional nonresorbable 4–0 stitches are used to secure the edge of the flap to the right atrium and the origin of the pulmonary artery.

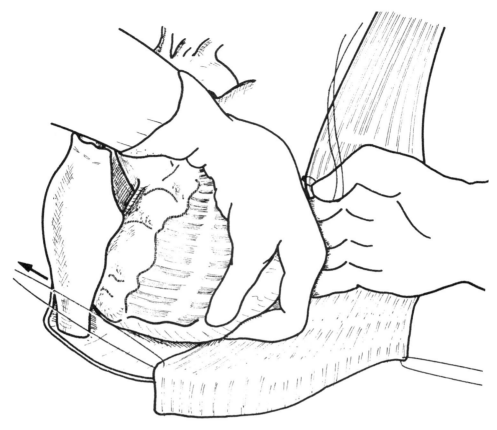

Figure 8.

The resorbable pilot sutures placed at the beginning of the positioning of the flap are left in place to reduce tension on the nonresorbable sutures.

Once the ventricular wrapping has been completed, a left paramedial vertical™ subcostal incision is made and a pocket is constructed behind the left rectus abdominalis fascia for the Cardiomyostimulator™ Pulse Train Generator (Fig. 11). The left side is preferred leaving the right side free in case a cholecystectomy is required in the future. The sensing electrodes and the stimulating electrodes are passed through the diaphragm to reach the stimulator to which they are connected. The aponeurosis and the skin are closed after a suction drain is placed in the pocket. The sternum is then closed with one drainage tube placed behind the sternum.

Anterior Wrapping

Whenever the right ventricle is predominantly affected, it is preferable to wrap it first. An anterior wrapping is also preferred by some authors (Magovern group) in biventricular failure based on the experimental findings that

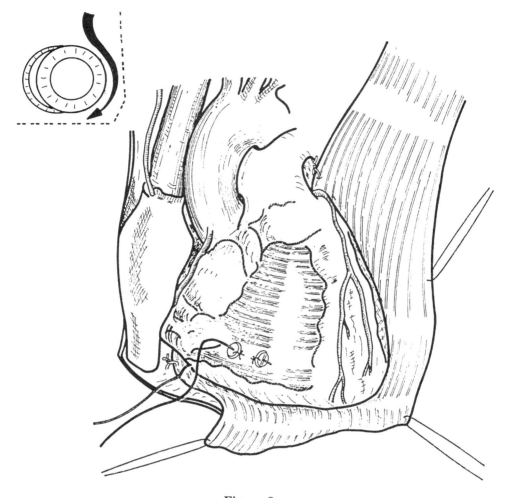

Figure 9.

anterior wrapping is more efficient. However, what is possible in dogs with normal size ventricles and rather long latissimus dorsi is rarely possible in humans if two dilated ventricles are to be covered, especially the left.

This modality raises in addition difficult problems of anterior wrapping muscle, stitching at the posterior aspect of the heart. In order to minimize these difficulties and to use the "no cardiac suture technique concept," the technique illustrated in Figure 12 has been developed.

A 15-cm long, 5-cm wide strip of pericardium is tailored. One of the smallest edges of the pericardial strip is sutured transversally to the posterior aspect of the muscle at the level of the left border of the heart. Sutures must be superficial so as not to compromise the vascularization of the muscle. The pericardial strip is positioned posterior to the heart while the muscle is po-

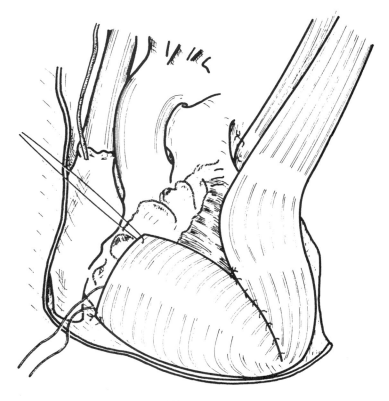

Figure 10.

sitioned anteriorly. The base of the muscle and the extremity of the pericardial strip are then sutured together at the diaphragmatic aspect of the heart.

Substitution Technique

The substitution technique is used whenever a tumor or large aneurysm is present and the remaining ventricular contractility is good. The latissimus dorsi mobilization and its transfer into the thorax are carried out in a similar manner. Likewise the lesions are approached through a median sternotomy. Atrial and aortic cannula are placed and connected to the extracorporeal circulation, which is necessary in this case. Whenever a tumor is present a large en bloc resection is carried out that may require either the removal and subsequent replacement of an atrioventricular valve or the bypass of an excised coronary artery. Whenever a large ventricular aneurysm is present, the aneurysm is resected at the limits of the scare with the exception of the interventricular septum (Fig. 13A). The defect left by the resection of the tumor or the aneurysm is closed using a glutaraldehyde-treated (0.6% glutaraldehyde in saline solution) autologous pericardial patch, the size of which is calculated

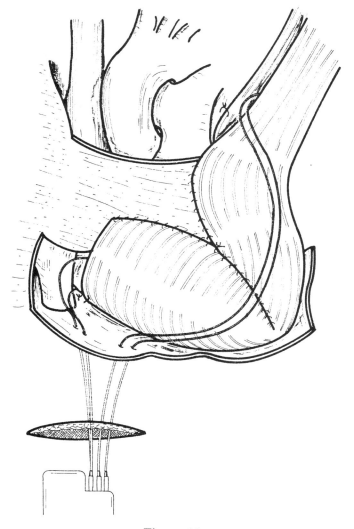

Figure 11.

to preserve an adequate volume to the ventricular cavity. In the case of an aneurysm, the circular patch is sutured to the septum so as to exclude most of the infarcted area according to the Jatene-Dor technique (Fig. 13B). The muscle flap is then sutured to the edge of the myocardial defect with 4–0 nonresorbable sutures (Fig. 13C).The upper part of the defect is sutured first to the deep surface of the muscle with superficial sutures so as not to impair muscle vascularization. The lower part of the defect is then sutured to the distal edge of the flap properly tailored to conform to the shape of the myocardial defect.

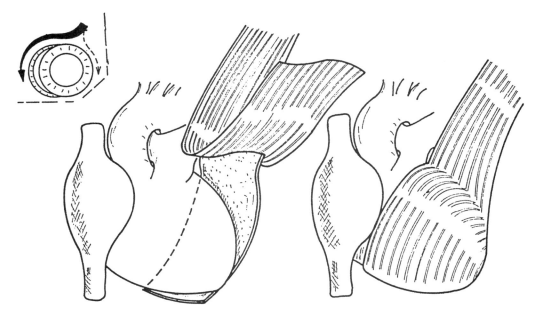

Figure 12.

Substitution and Reinforcement Technique

This modality is a combination of the two previously described techniques. The deep surface of the flap is sutured to the whole circumference of the myocardial defect and the remainder of the flap is wrapped around the two ventricles.

Electrical Stimulation of the Muscle

Cardiomyostimulator™ Pulse Train Generator

The development of the Cardiomyostimulator™ Pulse Train Generator required for this operation was the result of a 3-year cooperative effort between our research laboratory and Medtronic Europe. This programmable Cardiomyostimulator™ Pulse Train Generator (Medtronic Model 1005) is capable of delivering single impulses or a train of impulses at various frequencies (Fig. 14). It is also possible to vary the duration of stimulation for each cycle to allow at least a 75% recovery period. The stimulator is composed of two channels: a sensing channel that functions to detect cardiac activity and a pacing channel that stimulates muscle contraction based on the detection of QRS complexes. The sensing channel recently has been modified in order to improve R-wave signal detection in patients with diffuse myocardial disease.

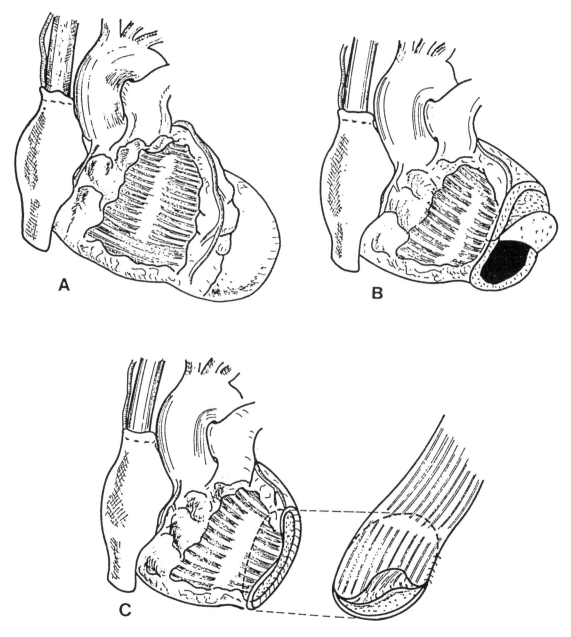

Figure 13.

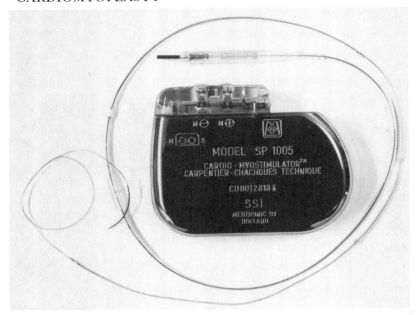

Figure 14.

An electronic circuit synchronizes the stimulation of the muscle with the cardiac activity. The ratio between cardiac contraction and muscle contraction can be modified 1:1, 2:1, 3:1. The delay between the cardiac signal and muscular contraction may also be programmed between 4 and 250 ms. In the event of atrioventricular block, the sensing channel automatically acts as a cardiac pacemaker. Additional interpretations are given in Chapter 9.

Electrodes

As shown by animal experiments, an efficient and diffuse muscle contraction is obtained by long wire electrodes passed through the muscular fibers at the point where the nerve branches and penetrates into the muscle. The stimulating electrodes made of platinum iridium alloy (Medtronic Model SP5520) are comprised of an adjustable length long wire so that contact can be established with the muscular mass only. Similar electrodes are used to detect the QRS complex on the ventricles. The sensing electrodes are comprised of a 4- to 5-cm wire that must be in full contact with the myocardium.

Stimulation Protocol

Skeletal muscle stimulation is initiated two weeks following cardiomyoplasty (Fig. 15). This delay allows postoperative skeletal muscle recovery (edema of the muscle and poor vascularization of its distal part are frequent

POST-OPERATIVE STIMULATION PROTOCOL

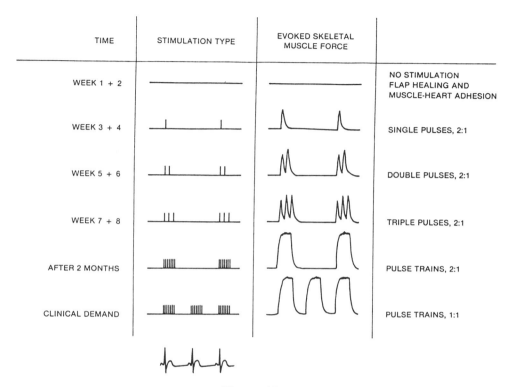

Figure 15.

immediately after latissimus dorsi mobilization) and adhesion of the muscle flap to the heart. The stimulation begins with single impulses for 2 weeks followed by double impulses (2 weeks) and subsequently trains of impulses (30-Hz burst, 6 pulses, pulse width 210 μsec) synchronized 2 to 1 with the cardiac cycle. A single impulse provokes a moderate muscle contraction. Trains of impulses provoke a temporal summation with recruitment of all muscle fibers and a strong contraction of the muscle. The duration of contraction is physiologically adapted to ventricular systole. There is a 25% stimulation time (duration of stimulation 185 ms) and a 75% recovery time (555 ms). The impulse amplitude is increased progressively to reach an average of 4 volts (±0.6). This cycle of stimulation together with the progressive stimulation protocol allow repetitive muscle contraction, without significant fatigue or muscle fiber degeneration. The full 1-to-1 or 1-to-2 stimulation with trains of impulses is initiated only 2 months after surgery. The mode 1 to 1 or 1 to 2 must be chosen based on the individual patient's comfort and activity and hemodynamic response as evaluated by echo Doppler. The timing of stimulation is essential to allow the muscle to contract only after mitral valve closure, and this is assessed by echocardiography.

This surgical technique together with the protocol of progressive sequential stimulation has provided the best functional results with reduced hospital mortality. (See Chapter 12.)

References

1. Carpentier A, Chachques JC, Grandjean PA: Transformation d'un muscle squelettique par stimulation sequentielle progressive en vue de son utilisation comme substitut myocardique. CR Acad Sc Paris 301:581, 1985.
2. Carpentier A, Chachques JC: Myocardial substitution with a stimulated skeletal muscle: first successful clinical case. Lancet 1:1267, 1985.
3. Carpentier A, Chachques JC: Latissimus dorsi cardiomyoplasty to increase cardiac output. In G Rabago, DA Cooley (eds): Heart Valve Replacement and Future Trends in Cardiac Surgery. Mount Kisco, NY, Futura Publishing Co, Inc, 1987, p 473.
4. Chacques JC, Grandjean PA, Carpentier A: Effect of latissimus dorsi dynamic cardiomyoplasty on ventricular function. Circulation 78 (Suppl 3):203–216, 1988.
5. Chacques JC, Mitz V, Hero M: Transsfert d'un muscle innerve sur le coeur. In G Nagalon, V Mitz (eds): Les Lambeaux Pedicules Musculaires. Paris, Masson, 1984, pp 5–6.

Chapter 9

Pulse Generator System for Dynamic Cardiomyoplasty

Pierre A. Grandjean

Dynamic cardiomyoplasty requires that the muscle grafted to the heart contract during the heart systolic phases.[1] This can be achieved by a system that detects heart contractions and electrically stimulates the grafted muscle to evoke its contraction during the ventricular periods. The "progressive sequential stimulation"[1] necessary to train the muscle before complete function can be obtained but requires a programmable system. A perfect management of the patient after operation is facilitated by a complete understanding of the function and feasibility of this system.

The implantable pulse generator, the Cardiomyostimulator™ Pulse Train Generator (Medtronic Model SP1005), which was developed to investigate this procedure,[2] is a programmable two-channel system that combines features found in dual-chamber cardiac pacing devices and neuromuscular stimulators, i.e., output synchronized to sensed or paced cardiac activity and burst of impulses for skeletal muscle stimulation (Fig. 1). It consists of a cardiac monitoring channel and a myostimulation channel, coordinated by a synchronization circuit (Table 1).

The heart monitor is composed of a sense amplifier that monitors the intrinsic heart rate and an output stage that paces the heart as soon as its rate drops below a programmed value. The sensing circuit reacts to the intrinsic deflection and slew rate of the ventricular signal collected by a myocardial or endocardial electrode .[2,3] The sensitivity of detection is programmable (0.6–2.5 mV) to ensure reliable QRS complex detection, even in depressed and dilated hearts (e.g., Chagas' disease). As in a demand pacemaker, a cardiac event can be sensed or initiated by the device in case of bradycardia.

The cardiac signal also triggers a synchronization circuit. A delay is then initiated after which the myostimulator outputs a burst of impulses to the muscle via a pair of leads. This synchronization delay is programmable to allow

From *Cardiomyoplasty* edited by Alain Carpentier, MD, PhD, Juan-Carlos Chachques, MD, and Pierre Grandjean, MS © 1991. Futura Publishing Inc., Mount Kisco, NY.

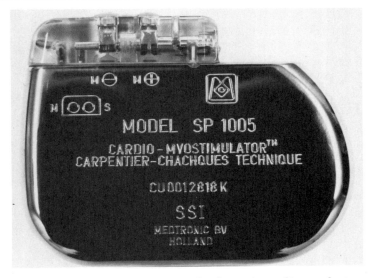

Figure 1. *The pulse generator for dynamic cardiomyoplasty.*

Table 1
SP1005 Pulse Generator: Main Characteristics

Cardiac Channel:	-Unipolar	
	-Lower rate:	40–120 PPM
	-Sensitivity:	.6–2.5 mV
	-Pulse amplitude:	2.5–5 V
	-Pulse width:	.05–1.5 ms
	-Refractory:	155–400 ms
Synchronization:	-Ratio: Mode I 1:1 when HR < 110 bpm	
	2:1 when 110 < HR < 200 bpm	
	Mode II 2:1 when HR < 110 bpm	
	3:1 when 110 < HR < 150 bpm	
	4:1 when 150 < HR < 200 bpm	
	-Delay: 4 − 250 ms	
Muscle Channel:	-Bipolar	
	-ON/OFF	
	-Pulse amplitude:	0–10.5 V
	-Pulse width:	.06–.5 ms
	-Frequency:	2–130 Hz
	-Max. burst duration:	185, 240 ms

Magnet mode: inhibits both channels
Power supply: lithium thionyl chloride batteries
Can material: titanium
Dimensions: 55 × 73 × 19 mm
Weight: 95 grams

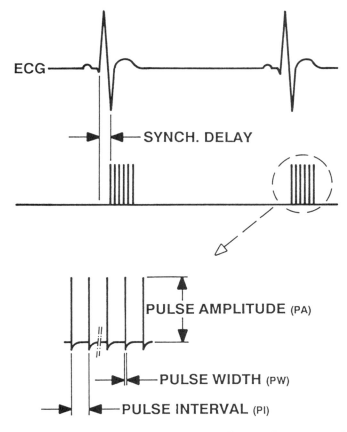

Figure 2. *Parameters of muscle stimulation synchronized on ventricular activity.*

optimal timing of the muscle contraction, which depends on heart conduction velocity, cardiac electrode placement, and heart/muscle complex reaction time (Fig. 2).

To allow for muscle adaptation to its new task, prevent its overuse (e.g., minimize muscle fatigue), and optimize cardiac benefits, the synchronization circuit has some additional safety features. These additional features allow different heart/muscle contractions ratios (2 modes) and prevent muscle stimulation at rates that are too high (110 or 55 contractions/min in mode I and II, respectively). This results in an automatic increase in heart/muscle contraction ratio whenever the heart rate exceeds the preset value (Fig. 3).

The myostimulator outputs balanced charge biphasic pulses. This type of pulse, while ensuring nerve fiber depolarization, prevents or minimizes the risk of neuromuscular tissue and electrode degradations by electrochemical processes.[4]

Pulse amplitude, pulse width, pulse interval, and burst duration are programmable. This high degree of flexibility in programming the myostimulator

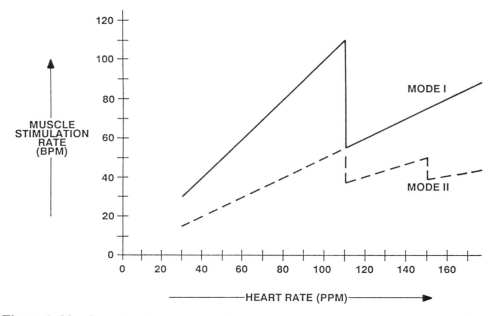

Figure 3. *Muscle contraction rate versus heart rate for two synchronization ratio modes.*

is necessary because of the way in which neuromuscular tissues react to electrical stimulation[4,5]. Altering the pulse amplitude or pulse width enables the gradation of the muscle force by varying the number of activated motor units (spatial recruitment, Fig. 4). The pulse interval (or frequency) grades the force by varying the rate of excitation of motor units (temporal summation, Fig. 5). As the stimulation frequency increases (or the pulse interval decreases), the force increases to reach a plateau at which the muscle contraction is smooth (fused contraction) (Fig. 6). Adjusting burst duration by increasing the number of pulses in the burst also enables evoked muscle force to be sustained over a longer period of time (Fig.6). For safety (e.g., to avoid muscle contraction extending during the diastolic phase), burst duration can be programmed at 185 and 240 ms and cannot exceed these values.

The main characteristics of the Cardiomyostimulator™ Pulse Train Generator are listed in Table 1. Parameters are programmable with the programming system shown in Figure 7. This system also enables interrogation and monitoring of the pulse generator status after implantation (e.g., review programmed parameters, check battery status, etc).

A Marker Channel™ feature facilitates determination of times of event detection (S) and start of muscle burst stimulation (P). "Marker signals" transmitted by the pulse generator and electrocardiogram signals collected by external leads can be printed by the programming system (Fig. 8). This feature is useful for determining whether or not a sensed event was generated by a heart contraction or by interference.

SPATIAL RECRUITMENT

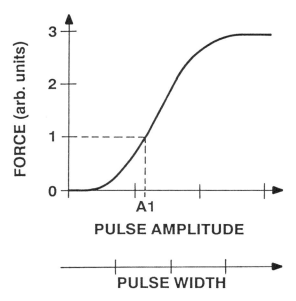

Figure 4. *Spatial recruitment: the evoked muscle force increases as the stimulus pulse amplitude or pulse width increases.*

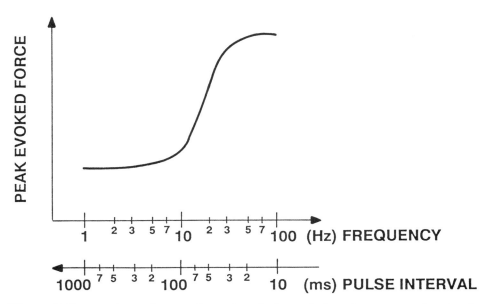

Figure 5. *Temporal recruitment: the peak evoked muscle force increases as the stimulus frequency increases (or the stimulus pulse interval decreases).*

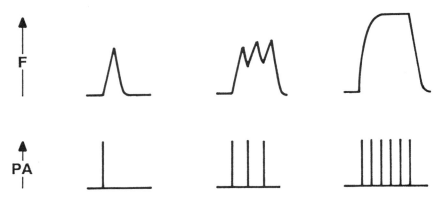

Figure 6. *Evoked muscle force and contraction duration adjustments by manipulation of stimulation parameters (number of pulses and pulse interval).*

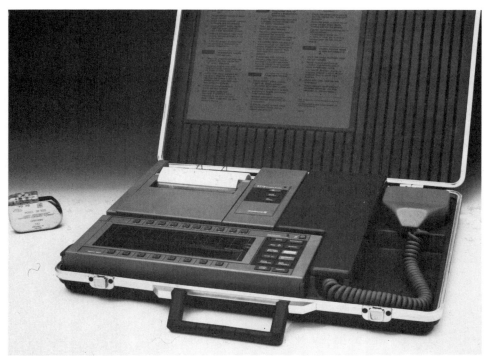

Figure 7. *Implantable pulse generator (left, Medtronic Model SP1005) and programming system (Medtronic Model 9710).*

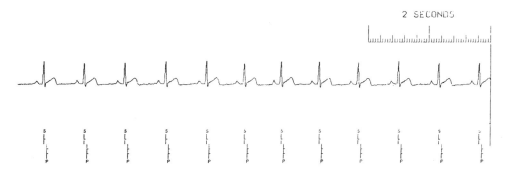

Figure 8. *Electrocardiogram and Marker Channel™ signals as printed by the programming system. The muscle channel is inhibited. S = time of sensed event; P = initiation time of muscle burst.*

Both channels of the pulse generator can be independently programmed "off." To allow for easy patient follow-up, the pulse generator can also be inhibited by application of a magnet.

Powered by high-current density lithium thionyl chloride batteries, this first generation implantable pulse generator is enclosed in a titanium can (55 x 73 x 19 mm) and weighs 95 grams. The lifetime depends on programmed parameters (pulse amplitude, pulse width, pulse interval, burst duration, synchronization mode, heart rate, electrode impedance). At standard values, it is estimated to be 24–30 months in the configuration described at the First Internation Workshop on Cardiomyoplasty.

Discussion

Currently used in cardiomyoplasty clinical investigations, this first generation implantable pulse generator, coupled to intramuscular leads (Medtronic Model SP5528) has provided a reliable means to stimulate the latissimus dorsi muscle in synchrony with heart contractions as used in the dynamic cardiomyoplasty procedure (Fig. 9)[3]. The stimulator parameter range facilitates the fine adjustments of the system needed for progressive muscle training after transfer to the heart ("progressive sequential" protocol[1]) and to regulate muscle contraction and its timing to optimize cardiac benefits.

The large range of muscle pacing parameters (pulse amplitude, pulse width) is also sufficient to deal with different types of implantable electrodes, or electrode positions, used in some neuromuscular stimulation investigations (e.g., intramuscular, nerve, epimysial electrodes).[6,7] In the cardiomyoplasty clinical investigation in the First International Workshop on Cardiomyoplasty, intramuscular leads (Medtronic Model SP5528[2]) are preferred due to their safety, reliability, and ease of placement.[8]

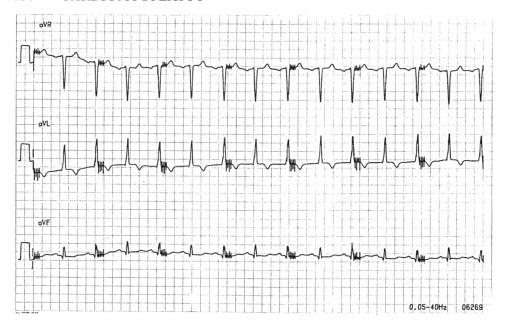

Figure 9. *Patient ECG recordings with the pulse generator programmed in mode II.*

References

1. Carpentier A, Chachques JC, Grandjean PA: Transformation d'un muscle squelet-tique par stimulation sequentielle progressive en vue de son utilisation comme sub-stitut myocardique. CR Acad Sc Paris 301:581, 1985.
2. Grandjean PA, Chachques JC, Carpentier A, et al: Implantable electronics and leads for muscular cardiac assistance. In RC-J Chiu (ed): Biomechanical Cardiac Assist: Cardiomyoplasty and Muscle Powered Devices. Mount Kisco, NY, Futura Publishing Co, 1986, p 103.
3. Grandjean PA, Herpers L, Smits K, et al: Performance of the Cardio-Myostimula-tor™ and intramuscular leads in the cardiomyoplasty procedure. In RC-J Chiu, I Bourgeois (eds): Transformed Skeletal Muscle for Cardiac Assist and Repair. Mount Kisco, NY, Futura Publishing Co, 1990, pp 231–240.
4. Mortimer JT: Motor prostheses. In VB Brooks (ed): Handbook of Physiology: the Nervous System. Bethesda, American Physiological Society, 1981, pp 155–187.
5. Guyton AC: Medical Physiology. Philadelphia, WB Saunders Co., 1980, chap 11.
6. Chiu RC-J, Bourgeois I (eds): Transformed Skeletal Muscle for Cardiac Assist and Repair. Mount Kisco, NY, Futura Publishing Co, 1990.
7. Hambrecht FT, Reswick JB(eds): Functional Electrical Stimulation: Application in Neural Prostheses. New York, Marcel Dekker, 1977.
8. Chachques JC, Chauvaud S, Carpentier A: Development of a nontiring stimulation of the latissimus dorsi flap used as a myocardial substitute. In H Thoma (ed): Pro-ceedings of the First Vienna International Workshop on Functional Electrical Stim-ulation. Vienna, 1983, pp 114–118.

Chapter 10

Postoperative Management

Juan-Carlos Chachques, Alain Carpentier

The postoperative management of cardiomyoplasty patients is particularly important to properly condition the muscle and to assess the efficiency of the operation.

Electrostimulation Protocol

Skeletal muscle can respond adaptively to increased functional demands such as those imposed by chronic electrical stimulation at slow rates.[1] A muscle that has been conditioned by progressive sequential stimulation has a greatly increased resistance to fatigue even at high rates and achieves a function similar to cardiac muscle.[2] Chronic skeletal muscle contraction in synchrony with ventricular systole is accomplished with specially designed pacing leads and a stimulator.

Electrodes

The two electrodes (Medtronic Model SP5528) used have been designed by one of us (JCC) to obtain optimal stimulation of the latissimus dorsi (LD) muscle, avoiding stimulation of other muscles. No mechanical or electrochemical adverse effects and no nerve damage have been found in patients with long-term implantation of these electrodes. Twitch threshold, full recruitment threshold, and impedance between electrodes are determined at the time of implantation.

The long-term synchronization between heart and LD muscle is assured by an intramyocardial sensing electrode (Medtronic model SP5548) that senses ventricular depolarization. Simultaneous contact with the epicardium and the myocardium allows reliable detection of the QRS complexes in patients suffering from diffused cardiomyopathies.

In ischemic disease that generally involves the LV, sensing electrodes are implanted into the RV wall. In patients with biventricular dilated cardiomyopathies, it is preferable to implant sensing electrodes into the LV wall.

From *Cardiomyoplasty* edited by Alain Carpentier, MD, PhD, Juan-Carlos Chachques, MD, and Pierre Grandjean, MS © 1991. Futura Publishing Inc., Mount Kisco, NY.

Pulse Generator

The systolic pulse generator used in the cardiomyoplasty procedure is a double-chamber stimulator that involves a sensing and a pacing channel (Cardiomyostimulator™ Pulse Train Generator, Medtronic Model SP1005). An electronic circuit synchronizes stimulation of muscle contraction with cardiac activity after a programmed delay (4-250 ms) and determines the heart:muscle synchronization ratio (i.e., 1:1, 2:1, 3:1). In the event of atrioventricular block, the sensing channel automatically acts as a cardiac pacemaker. The pulse generator programming is performed by radiofrequency telemetry. Battery life can be monitored by the same procedure. Pulse generator inhibition is possible by using an external magnet.

Postoperative Stimulation Protocol

Unlike the heart, which is an electrical and mechanical syncytium, skeletal muscle is modulated by the number and rate at which fibers are activated. A single electrical stimulus resulting in a single muscle twitch does not normally generate sufficient force to augment cardiac function. However, rapid repetitive stimuli delivered before the muscles fiber completes its relaxation results in mechanical summation until fusion occurs, which causes the muscle to generate substantial force.[3]

The latissimus dorsi muscle flap (LDMF) is left undisturbed for 2 to 3 weeks after cardiomyoplasty before gradual exercise is begun. This delay is necessary for the development of LDMF collateral circulation and to allow formation of adhesions among the heart, muscle flap, and pericardium. The electrostimulation protocol is not rigid and fixed, but instead is designed to consider the operation performed, the extent of the LD muscle fixation over the heart, the patient's postoperative course, the response of ventricular function to pharmacotherapy, and the amount of disuse skeletal muscle atrophy present.[4] (See Chapter 8 for details.)

The protocol for postoperative sequential and progressive skeletal muscle electrostimulation begins with single impulses and ultimately culminates in a train of impulses (burst frequency: 30 Hz) coordinated with the cardiac cycle (Fig. 1). Pulse generator activation is begun under electrocardiographic and echocardiographic monitoring. The impulse amplitude is increased gradually until a moderate contraction of the LD muscle is palpated over its extrathoracic segment. The mean skeletal muscle pulse amplitude used in our series of 20 patients was 4.1 ± 0.6 V (30-Hz burst, 6 pulses, pulse width 210 μsec.).

Patients have shown a remarkable tolerance to chronic LD muscle contraction. No cardiac arrhythmias, pain, or discomfort have been observed as a result of skeletal muscle electrostimulation. Hospitalization is not required during the training period. Most of the patients were chronically stimulated using burst stimulation with a heart-to-muscle contraction ratio of 2:1.

Method of Follow-up

The postoperative course of cardiomyoplasty patients is influenced by their preoperative status, co-existing diseases, and type of operation performed. The

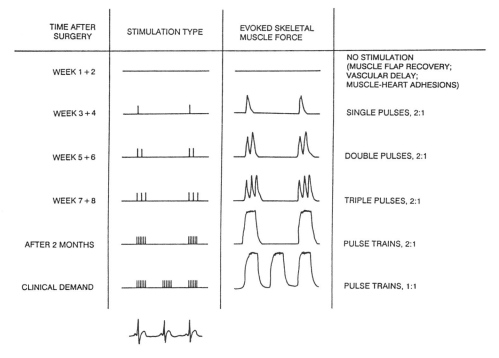

TIME AFTER SURGERY	STIMULATION TYPE	EVOKED SKELETAL MUSCLE FORCE	
WEEK 1 + 2			NO STIMULATION (MUSCLE FLAP RECOVERY; VASCULAR DELAY; MUSCLE-HEART ADHESIONS)
WEEK 3 + 4			SINGLE PULSES, 2:1
WEEK 5 + 6			DOUBLE PULSES, 2:1
WEEK 7 + 8			TRIPLE PULSES, 2:1
AFTER 2 MONTHS			PULSE TRAINS, 2:1
CLINICAL DEMAND			PULSE TRAINS, 1:1

Figure 1. *Postoperative stimulation protocol. The LD muscle is electrically conditioned over a 6-week period, starting generally on the 14th postoperative day. After the protocol is started, stimulation is continuous 24 h/day.*

reinforcement technique (latissimus dorsi muscle wrapped around ventricles for ischemic or dilated cardiomyopathies) does not necessitate cardiopulmonary bypass in the absence of associated pathologies and therefore eliminates the specific complications of extracorporeal circulation. The substitution technique (partial replacement of the ventricular wall after aneurysm or tumor resections) add occasional problems of ventricular compliance to the inconvenience of extracorporeal circulation. Since this technique requires the use of a pericardial patch to protect the muscle from high pressure blood infiltration, heparin is indicated for a period of 10 days to avoid intraventricular thrombosis.

The evaluation of the efficacy of a cardiomyoplasty is based on functional results (i.e., functional class, quality of life, professional activity) and paraclinical investigations. Not only is the comparison between pre- and postoperative findings important but also the studies done both at rest and during exercise.

The effect of LDMF dynamic contractions is evaluated by studies comparing assisted and nonassisted cycles (heart:LDMF stimulation ratio 2:1, 3:1) or by comparing the hemodynamic profile with the pulse generator in the ON and OFF modes (magnet mode). Some drugs, principally psycholeptics and psychotropics, have adverse effects on the amount of force a skeletal muscle can generate during contraction, and their use should be limited after cardiomyoplasty.

Postoperative evaluation includes ECG, posterior-anterior and lateral chest X ray, 2D and Doppler echocardiography (transcutaneous or transesophageal), technetium 99m multigated scan at rest and during exercise, Holter monitoring, oxygen uptake during exercise (including lactic acid quantification), and respiratory function tests. These studies are performed every 4 months during the first postoperative year and twice a year thereafter.

At one year, a CT scan and catheterization with ventriculography are obtained. CT scanning and ultrafast computed tomography (Imatron) evaluates the LD muscle wrapping, segmental contraction of ventricles (identification of asynergic areas) and the ventricular systolic and diastolic volumes. Catheterization and ventriculography are performed to determine cardiac index, LV end-systolic and end-diastolic pressures and volumes, ejection fraction, and ventricular geometrical shape.

The clinical entity of diastolic dysfunction is heterogeneous and difficult to define numerically. Diastolic itself is a complex set of separate but interrelated processes. Although all indexes of diastolic functions have limitations (isovolumic relaxation, early diastolic rapid filling, diastasis, atrial contraction, and end diastole)[5] these indexes serve as a useful framework in the evaluation of a cardiomyoplasty. Postoperative studies show that cardiomyoplasty limits the dilatation of the heart, avoiding regional inhomogeneities during diastole.

The efficacy of electrostimulation is evaluated by muscle contractile response. When the latissimus dorsi muscle is into the chest, its force of contraction is not easy to quantify. Dynamic muscle contraction can be detected by palpation in the area of the second rib window where the LD muscle has been reattached. Each LD muscle stimulation results in a palpable contraction. LDMF contraction within the chest can also be monitored by echocardiography (percutaneous or transesophageal). The role of electromyography in following LD muscle function postoperatively is still not clearly defined. Future studies will elucidate the feasibility and utility of postoperative intrathoracic electromyography.

Current clinical experience shows that almost all cardiomyoplasty patients are clinically improved or stabilized in the long term. Episodes of acute heart failure (pulmonary edema) are eliminated and the number of arrhythmias is reduced. Moreover, overall pharmacological support generally is reduced after cardiomyoplasty. LV function gradually improves up to the sixth postoperative month. This is most likely due to (1) the gradual increase in the LD muscle resistance to fatigue, and (2) better matching of the cardiac output to the demands of the contracting muscle flap and beneficial effects that the contracting muscle has on LV function.

Postoperative Complications

Following is a description of several complications that can affect the course of a cardiomyoplasty.

Ischemic and Bacterial Myonecrosis

Diabetes and advanced age are important risk factors in latissimus dorsi postoperative myonecrosis. Low cardiac output and inotropic drugs (peripheral vasoconstrictors) contribute to this complication. Ischemic myonecrosis generally is associated with torsion, traction, or surgical hematoma of the LD muscle pedicle; excessive use of electrocautery during mobilization of the LDMF; or muscle compression at the second rib window. Bacterial myonecrosis usually is associated with septic mediastinis. The presence of blood, edema, necrotic tissue, or foreign bodies contributes to the development of regional opportunistic infection.

Symptoms of myonecrosis have been described in plastic surgery. They include intoxication, mental confusion, irritability or apathy, marked tachycardia, tachypnea, sweating, pallor, and lack of coordination. Very high serum creatine kinase (CK) levels may have some predictive value.[6] We have not seen this complication in our practice although CK increase in some patients suggested that at least some localized necrosis may have occurred.

Functional Impairment of the Shoulder and Arm

The rotation to the LD muscle into the chest cavity caused little functional impairment of the shoulder and arm. The contractions of the LD muscle during the conditioning period and later did not affect the motion of the upper limb, and patients did not report discomfort (Fig. 2). It is important to emphasize

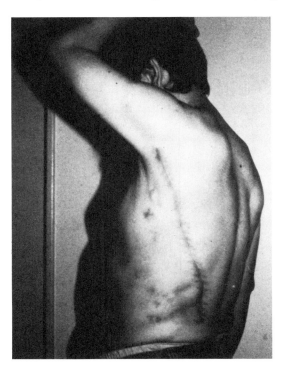

Figure 2. *The transfer of the LD muscle into the chest and its electrostimulation does not cause functional impairment to the upper limb.*

that the LD muscle humeral tendon must be divided during surgery. Specially tailored exercises of the left upper limb are indicated after the second postoperative week.

Dorsal Subcutaneous Seroma

Between the 8th and the 20th postoperative days a seroma frequently occurs in the area of LD muscle dissection. The measures to prevent seroma formation are rigorous intraoperative hemostasis, placement of suction drains, and suturing the cutaneous flaps to the chest wall. Currently we are studying the efficacy of fibrin glue to promote adhesions between the skin and the chest wall.

Seroma usually does not require special care and only compression is recommended until spontaneous reabsorbtion occurs. Nevertheless, in some cases it was necessary to reinsert subcutaneous drains. Secondary wound infection and skin necrosis rarely have occurred.

Cardiomyostimulator™ Pulse Train Generator Pocket Infection

To reduce the risk of pulse generator pocket infection, its implantation is always performed beneath the abdominis muscle fascia, far from the pericardial, pleural, and wound drains. In the event of infection, one can try to preserve the leads and the implanted stimulator by local antiseptic irrigation and drainage and systematic antibacterial therapy. Removal of the device is performed if sensing or pacing function is compromised, an abscess develops around the leads, or the patient develops signs of systemic sepsis. The majority of pocket infections are secondary to either *Staphylococcus aureus* or *Staphylococcus epidermidis*. The use of antibiotics in the perioperative period reduces the incidence of surgical wound infections. For maximum effectiveness, the antibiotic should be given prior to incision.[7]

Respiratory Failure

The LD muscle occupies approximately 10% of the hemithorax volume.[8] Nevertheless, to prevent early postoperative ventilatory problems in the intensive care unit, all patients undergo 2 weeks of preoperative respiratory therapy (incentive spirometry, deep breathing and coughing exercises), and intensive pulmonary therapy must be continued after surgery. Major respiratory insufficiency is a contraindication to cardiomyoplasty.

Cardiac Arrhythmias

The hearts of patients that undergo cardiomyoplasty are prone to the development of arrhythmias. Dilated cardiomyopathies and resection of ventricular aneurysms are especially prone to tachyarrhythmias. If indicated, postoperative cardioversion can be performed either transcutaneously or by transesophageal electrode. A risk of pulse generator damage may exist depending on cardioversion parameters and electrode positions. Heart block is uncommon following the cardiomyoplasty procedure. In these cases, the pulse generator acts as both a cardiac and muscle stimulator.

Heart Failure

Postoperative cardiac tamponade rarely is seen since the pericardium is left opened and the left mediastinal pleura is always incised. However, in order to avoid blood collection between the muscular flap and the heart, this virtual space should not be hermetically sutured.

The hemodynamic benefits of cardiomyoplasty do not begin for several weeks due to the time period needed for postoperative muscle recovery and training, therefore before patients are selected for this procedure their residual ventricular function must be taken into account.[9-11] Inotropic drugs, intra-aortic balloon counterpulsation, or other types of ventricular assist devices can be useful to support cardiac function during the immediate postoperative period. Patients who are unstable hemodynamically or on inotropic drug support prior to surgery are not candidates for cardiomyoplasty. Furthermore, patients with severe biventricular heart failure or severe pulmonary artery hypertension are at an extremely high risk for morbidity and mortality postoperatively.

External Lung Herniation

In two patients with chronic bronchoemphysema, we have observed intermittent lung herniation through the area of the second rib resection during fits of coughing. Both patients tolerated this well and did not require further intervention.

Postoperative Cholecystitis

In three patients, we observed postoperative cholecystitis. Two of these patients required cholecystectomy. Because of this experience we now implant the pulse generator in the left upper abdominal quadrant, leaving the right upper quadrant free.

References

1. Salmons S, Henriksson J: The adaptative response of skeletal muscle to increased use. Muscle Nerve 4:94, 1981.
2. Carpentier A, Chachques JC, Grandjean PA: Transformation d'un muscle squelettique par stimulation sequentielle progressive en vue de son utilisation comme substitut myocardique. CR Acad Sc Paris 301:581, 1985.

 3. Acker MA, Anderson WA, Hammond RL, et al: Skeletal muscle ventricles in circulation. J Thorac Cardiovasc Surg 94:163, 1987.
 4. Wiener DH, Fink LI, Maris J, et al: Abnormal skeletal muscle bioenergetics during exercise in patients with heart failure: role of reduced muscle blood flow. Circulation 73:1127, 1986.
 5. Lew WYW: Evaluation of left ventricular diastolic function. Circulation 79:1393, 1989.
 6. Ahrenholz DH: Necrotizing soft-tissue infections. Surg Clin North Am 68:199, 1988.
 7. Young EJ, Sugarman B: Infections in prosthetic devices. Surg Clin North Am 68:167, 1988.
 8. Shesol BV, Clarke JS: Intrathoracic application of the Latissimus Dorsi musculocutaneous flap. Plast Reconstr Surg 66:842, 1980.
 9. Hammermeister KE, Chikos PM, Fisher L, et al: Relationship of cardiothoracic ratio and plain film heart volume to late survival. Circulation 59:89, 1979.
10. Franciosa JA, Wilen M, Ziesche S, et al: Survival in men with severe chronic left ventricular failure due to either coronary heart disease or idiopathic dilated cardiomyopathy. Am J Cardiol 51:831, 1983.
11. Pfeffer MA, Pfeffer JM: Ventricular enlargement and reduced survival after myocardial infarction. Circulation 75 (Suppl 4):93, 1987.

Chapter 11

Surgical Technique at Allegheny General Hospital

George J. Magovern, Race L. Kao, Ignacio Y. Christlieb*

In spite of a recent continuing decline in the death rate from cardiovascular diseases, there is still a steady increase in patients who suffer chronic heart failure. Sudden or progressive failure of the heart causes the early death of many persons who are otherwise healthy. Despite significant advances in medical management, the mortality rate is more than 50% within five years after diagnosis of congestive heart failure.[1,2] Dynamic cardiomyoplasty involves the use of an electrically stimulated skeletal muscle positioned on the heart to correct a cardiac defect and to improve circulation (see ref. 3 for review). In addition to an artificial heart or cardiac transplantation, dynamic cardiomyoplasty offers a permanent circulatory support for end-stage heart failure patients without the limitations of tissue rejection, donor shortages, prohibitive costs, and complex energy sources.

Experimental Studies at Allegheny-Singer Research Institute

Experimental studies using sheep of the Dorsett-Merino cross stock with a body weight of 72 ± 3 kg and mongrel dogs weighing 25 to 35 kg were the basis of our clinical experience. The animals were anesthetized with Pentothal (25 mg/kg) before preparation for sterile surgical procedures. Alepromazine (15 mg) and atropine (0.5 mg) were given to the sheep to control bronchial, gastric, and salivary secretions. All animals received humane care in compliance with the "Principles of Laboratory Animal Care" and "Guide for the Care and Use of Laboratory Animals." The electrocardiogram was monitored through a lead on each leg with arterial, venous, and ventricular pressure lines connected to a Hewlett Packard 8890B System for recording. A Swan-Ganz thermodilution catheter was used to measure cardiac output and pressures. Since increasing cardiac output in a dog with a normal heart and cir-

* With the cooperation of FR Heckler and SB Park.
From *Cardiomyoplasty* edited by Alain Carpentier, MD, PhD, Juan-Carlos Chachques, MD, and Pierre Grandjean, MS © 1991. Futura Publishing Inc., Mount Kisco, NY.

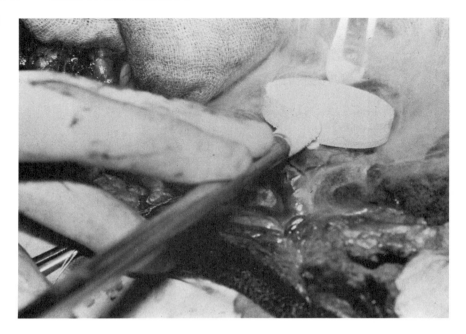

Figure 1. *Cryoinjury of the heart.*

culatory regulating system by compressing the ventricular wall is impractical, 3 mg/kg propranolol was infused intravenously to induce temporary heart failure for the functional study.

After exposing the heart following a sternotomy, a cryoprobe of 5-cm diameter made of copper alloy cooled to −160°C by internally circulating liquid nitrogen was used to induce cryoinjury of the heart. Following administration of heparin (2,000 units) and lidocaine (50 mg), the selected area of myocardium was frozen by applying the cryoprobe for three minutes. (Fig. 1). The frozen heart muscle thawed in a few minutes and showed a well-defined area with cyanotic color and hypokinesis. Edema and bulging of the cryoinjured area with nonviable myocytes, marked vascular congestion, focal extravasation of red blood cells, and small numbers of infiltrating neutrophils and macrophages were observed. The inflammatory process gradually subsided in 4 to 6 weeks with fibrous scar formation at the cryoinjured site. The custom-made pericardial pouch sutured to the remaining rim of the resected scar tissue formed the ventricular aneurysm (Fig. 2) with paradoxical movement against each heart beat. Color Doppler studies revealed the compression of the muscle flap on the aneurysmal sack. The benefit of different skeletal muscle fiber orientations using the aneurysm model is under current investigation.

Based upon our earlier experience, sequential stimulation (either single or burst) can achieve the transformation of skeletal muscle fibers. The significant increase in type I fibers and succinate dehydrogenase-positive fibers in animals that were followed for 12 months are shown in Figure 3. Ultra-

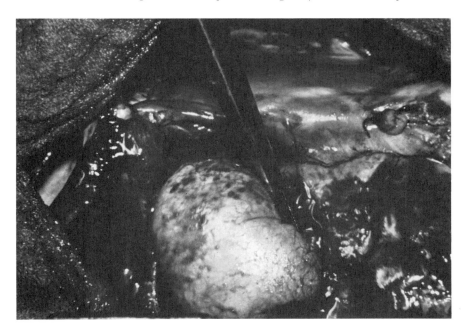

Figure 2. *Ventricular aneurysm created by the pericardial pouch.*

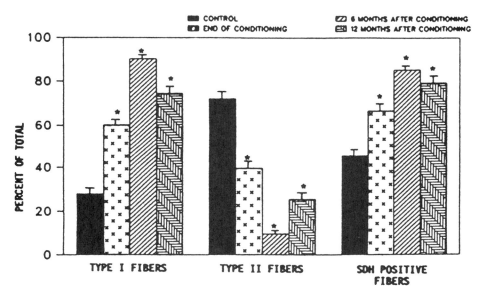

Figure 3. *Changes in muscle fibers after chronic electric stimulation. *-Significantly different from control with p <.01.*

structural evaluations reveal the typical increase of Z-band width and mito-chondrial content with the decrease of T-system and sarcoplasmic reticulum. For one patient (the third one in our series), the latissimus dorsi muscle had been conditioned for 10 weeks before the dynamic cardiomyoplasty procedure. During the surgical procedure, muscle biopsies were obtained, and the trans-formation of fiber types was documented by histochemical and ultrastructural evaluations.[5]

Clinical Experience at Allegheny General Hospital

At Allegheny General Hospital, seven patients (3 females and 4 males) suffering refractory congestive heart failure were subjected to dynamic car-diomyoplasty procedures. Age ranged from 45 to 65 years (mean ± SE = 56 ± 3), and ejection fractions ranged from 19% to 38% (mean ± SE = 26 ± 2) before surgery. The patient data are summarized in Table 1. The left latissimus dorsi muscle with its intact neurovascular bundle was applied over the ven-tricular wall to repair a myocardial defect and/or to improve cardiac function.

The muscle was dissected free from all insertions with complete preser-vation of the thoracodorsal neurovascular bundle. After resection of a portion of the second or third rib, the muscle flap was internalized into the thoracic cavity with the freed humeral tendinous end sutured to the tissue surrounding the resected rib. The skeletal muscle was used to partially cover the ventricles in four patients (Fig. 4a) and to completely wrap around the heart in three patients (Fig. 4c).

Table 1
Summary of Patient Data

	Yes	No
Diffused coronary artery disease	6	1
Ventricular aneurysm	4	3
Aneurysmectomy	3	4
Coronary artery bypass graft	3	4

Pulse Generators and Leads Used

Two types of commercially available cardiac pacemakers and one type of FDA-approved investigational pulse generator have been used in the clinical studies. Two patients received Symbios™ (Medtronic Model 7206), two pa-tients received Delta™ 925 (Cardiac Pacemakers, Inc. [CPI]), and three pa-tients were expected to receive Medtronic Model SP1005 as pulse generators.

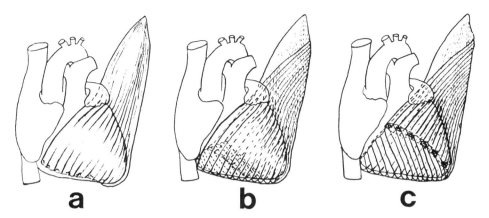

Figure 4. *Different ways to wrap the muscle flap on the heart. a = partial anterior wrap; b = complete anterior wrap; c = complete posterior wrap.*

One 4315 sutureless myocardial lead from CPI was placed on the right ventricle for sensing in all patients except the first one who received two 4951 sutureless atrial/ventricular leads from Medtronic on the right atrium. Medtronic Model 4951, 6917, or SP5528, or the CPI 4315 or 4260 leads were used to stimulate the latissimus dorsi muscle.

Surgical Procedures

As shown in Table 1, the first three patients were subjected to aneurysmectomy. In the first case, a part of the aneurysmal wall was left intact to avoid the reduction of left ventricular size. The second and third patients had standard repair, and in all three patients the left latissimus dorsi muscle covered the ventricular wall, which included the site of the aneurysmectomy. Patients 4, 5, and 6 had coronary artery bypass grafts. The first four patients had the anterior wrap of the muscle flap that covered a major portion of both ventricles (Fig. 4a). The last three patients had a posterior wrap with the muscle flap covering the entire ventricle (Fig. 1c).

From the clinical experience at Allegheny General Hospital, it is possible to extend the cardiomyoplasty procedure to combined aneurysmectomy and coronary artery bypass as well as to primary cardiomyopathy. Since skeletal muscle contracts primarily in the direction of its fiber orientation, how to utilize this contractile force to maximize the cardiac output of an ailing heart is one of our major concerns. In experimental animals with fully conditioned latissimus dorsi muscle after dynamic cardiomyoplasty, the anteriorly wrapped muscle (Fig. 4b) provided significant benefit in hemodynamic performance under propranolol-induced temporary heart failure. However, a similar improvement in our clinical cases cannot be proved due to variations in surgical procedure and the small number of patients.

Complications in Clinical Cases

Of the seven patients, the third and sixth patients died from different causes. The third patient had his muscle flap preconditioned with a neurological pulse generator (Itrel[TM] 7420) before the cardiomyoplasty procedure. Dissection of the muscle flap during the second operation was more difficult, and a large seroma formed at the skeletal muscle site, after the procedure the seroma drained for three weeks. The infection most likely started at the flap site and lead to the loss of latissimus dorsi muscle function. The patient died of a fatal arrhythmia from a heart encased in an infected and degenerated muscle flap.

The second mortality was directly related to uncontrollable oozing from the skeletal muscle site that also bled into the chest cavity. Multiple blood components and open packing were required to control the bleeding. The patient developed hypotension with low systemic vascular resistance and eventually died of multiple organ failure before skeletal muscle conditioning was initiated. These results prompted us to perform the operating procedures in two separate stages. For the seventh patient, the left latissimus dorsi was freed from all but the humeral and iliac crest insertions. The proximal and distal pacing electrodes were placed with the neurovascular bundle carefully preserved. The patient was allowed to recover for 48 hours before wrapping the muscle around the heart. The muscle was slightly edematous, but otherwise healthy. Most importantly, hematoma and seroma did not occur, and the postoperative recovery was significantly improved.

Discussion

Skeletal muscle is an extremely heterogenous tissue comprised of different myofibers with variable patterns of assembly. The plasticity of skeletal muscle that adapts to new physiological demands is well established.[6-8] Muscle transformation during chronic electric stimulation involving changes in contractile proteins, increases in capillary supply, and expansion of oxidative capacity was observed in this study as reported by several other investigators.[8-10]

Electrically conditioned skeletal muscle has been used to power cardiac assist devices,[11,12] to construct skeletal muscle ventricles,[13] and to augment heart function directly[14,15] in experimental animals. Clinically, latissimus dorsi muscle has been utilized to reconstruct the ventricle after excision of cardiac tumor[16] or ventricular aneurysm,[17] to assist dyskinetic ventricle,[18-20] and to benefit patients with dilated cardiomyopathy.[5,21,22]

From our experience, dynamic cardiomyoplasty significantly improved ventricular wall motion and stabilized the septal wall to correct the paradoxical movement. Cardiac output and ejection fraction were clearly increased, especially during exercise. Further dilatation of the ventricles was prevented, and an increase in myocardial blood supply was possible.

The clinical experience with seven patients over almost a 4-year period has shown a number of important improvements in the surgical technique of dynamic cardiomyoplasty, including:

1. conditioning of the skeletal muscle,
2. placement of the electrodes and pulse generator,
3. method of wrapping the latissimus dorsi around the heart, and
4. staging of the procedure in two operations.

Unfortunately, with only seven patients, no two operations were identical. This is mainly due to the fact that dynamic cardiomyoplasty is still in its experimental phase and an established protocol for surgical procedures and pacing equipment is not available. There is an advantage in that improvements from laboratory results can be integrated immediately into clinical practice. However, the inability to statistically compare different surgical techniques between patients is a major disadvantage.

In our opinion, the following are important technical points in dynamic cardiomyoplasty:

1. Free the humeral attachment of the skeletal muscle: this procedure not only provides more usable muscle to wrap around the ventricle but also avoids accidental dislocation of intercostal attachments.

2. Improve the pulse generator and electrodes: the ideal cardiomyostimulator is not available, and improvement in pacing leads is absolutely necessary.

3. Orient the muscle with proper fiber direction: with the skeletal muscle contracting mainly in the direction of its fiber orientation, this can be a primary factor in maximizing the cardiac output for each patient by dynamic cardiomyoplasty.

4. Perform the operative procedures in two stages: by freeing the latissimus dorsi 48 hours before wrapping it around the heart, hematoma and seroma can be prevented with significant improvement in postoperative recovery.

References

1. Smith WM: Epidemiology of congestive heart failure. Am J Cardiol 55:3A, 1985.
2. Dollery CT, Corr L: Drug treatment of heart failure. Br Heart J 54:234, 1985.
3. Chiu RC-J (ed): Biomechanical Cardiac Assist: Cardiomyoplasty and Muscle-Powered Devices. Mount Kisco, NY: Futura Publishing Co, Inc, 1986.
4. Dubowitz V, Brooke MH: Muscle Biopsy: A Modern Approach. Philadelphia, PA: W.B. Saunders Co, 1973.
5. Magovern GJ, Heckler FR, Park SB, et al: Paced skeletal muscle for dynamic cardiomyoplasty. Ann Thorac Surg 45:614, 1988.
6. Pette D (ed): Plasticity of Muscle. Berlin, New York, de Gruyter, 1980.
7. Faulkner JA, Carlson BM: Skeletal muscle regeneration: a historical perspective. Fed Proc 45:1454, 1986.
8. Carraro U (ed): Sarcomeric and Non-Sarcomeric Muscles: Basic and Applied Research Prospects for the 90's. Padova, Italy, Unipress Padova, 1988.
9. Brister S, Fradet G, Dewar M, et al: Transforming skeletal muscle for myocardial assist: a feasibility study. Can J Surg 28:341, 1985.
10. Mannion JD, Bitto T, Hammond RL, et al: Histochemical and fatigue characteristics of conditioned canine latissimus dorsi muscle. Circ Res 58:298, 1986.

11. Acker MA, Hammond RL, Mannion JD, et al: Skeletal muscle as the potential power source for a cardiovascular pump: assessment in vivo. Science 236:324, 1987.
12. Kochamba G, Desrosiers C, Dewar M, et al: The muscle-powered dual-chamber counterpulsator: rheologically superior implantable cardiac assist device. Ann Thorac Surg 45:620, 1988.
13. Mannion JD, Acker MA, Hammond RL, et al: Power output of skeletal muscle ventricles in circulation: acute studies. Circulation 76:155, 1987.
14. Chachques JC, Grandjean PA, Tommasi JJ, et al: Dynamic cardiomyoplasty: a new approach to assist chronic myocardial failure. Life Support Sys 5:323, 1987.
15. Dewar M, Walsh G, Abraham R, et al: Left ventricular full-thickness cardiomyoplasty with pericardial neoendocardium: experimental development of a surgical procedure. Ann Thorac Surg 44:618, 1987.
16. Carpentier A, Chachques JC: Myocardial substitution with a stimulated skeletal muscle: first successful clinical case. Lancet 1:1267, 1985.
17. Magovern GJ, Park SB, Magovern GJ Jr, et al: Latissimus dorsi as a functioning synchronously paced muscle component in the repair of a left ventricular aneurysm. Ann Thorac Surg 41:116, 1986.
18. Carpentier A, Chachques JC: Latissimus dorsi cardiomyoplasty to increase cardiac output. In G Rabago, DA Cooley (eds): Heart Valve Replacement and Future Trends in Cardiac Surgery. Mount Kisco, NY, Futura Publishing Co, Inc, 473, 1987.
19. Magovern GJ, Heckler FR, Park SB, et al: Paced latissimus dorsi used for dynamic cardiomyoplasty of left ventricular aneurysms. Ann Thorac Surg 44:379, 1987.
20. Dumcius A, Salcius K, Giedraitis S, et al: Myoventriculoplasty with the use of programmed, physiologically controlled electroneurostimulation. J Thorac Cardiovasc Surg 97:636, 1989.
21. Chachques JC, Grandjean P, Schwartz K, et al: Effect of latissimus dorsi dynamic cardiomyoplasty on ventricular function. Circulation 78(suppl III):III-203, 1988.
22. Molteni L, Almada H, Ferreira R: Synchronously stimulated skeletal muscle graft for left ventricular assistance: case report. J Thorac Cardiovasc Surg 97:439, 1989.

Chapter 12

Hôpital Broussais Clinical Experience

I. Patient Selection
Alain Carpentier

II. Preassist Period
Bernard Abry, Alain Carpentier

III. Postassist Period
Serban Mihaileanu, Juan-Carlos Chachques

I. Patient Selection

From January 1985 to June 1989, 20 patients suffering from severe heart failure were operated on at Broussais. For ethical reasons, the majority were selected from patients who had been proposed for heart transplantation but in whom pretransplant investigations showed one or several contraindications.

Etiology

In the majority of the cases the cause of heart failure was either chronic myocardial ischemia or nonobstructive cardiomyopathy (Table 1).

The 12 patients with heart failure of **ischemic origin** had suffered several myocardial infarctions. They were all beyond the possibility of complete myocardial revascularization. In three patients, who still had one coronary artery amenable to bypass, i.e., the left marginal in two patients and the anterior descending in one patient, revascularization of these arteries was thought to be useful to slow the evolution of the underlying disease and to prevent a recurrent myocardial infarction. In this ischemic group, six patients had a global dilatation of the heart and six had an extensive anteroapical left ventricular aneurysm. Of the six patients with a dilated heart, one had a mitral valve insufficiency and one a mitral and tricuspid valve insufficiency. Of the

Table 1	
Etiology	
Ischemic Heart Disease	*12*
With aneurysm	6
Dilated heart	6
Cardiomyopathy	*6*
Idiopathic	5
Valvular	1
Tumor	*2*

five patients with a left ventricular aneurysm, four had a reduced contractility of the remaining myocardium and two had an exceptionally large aneurysm requiring a large patching of the ventricle in order to preserve an adequate residual diastolic volume of the left ventricle.

Five patients suffered idiopathic cardiomyopathy. Two of them suffered from severe insulin-dependent diabetes, and one had had a full protocol of irradiation for Hodgkin's disease 5 years before cardiomyoplasty.

One patient had a valvular cardiomyopathy of rheumatic origin that did not improve significantly after an aortic valve replacement and a prosthetic ring mitral valve reconstruction performed $1\frac{1}{2}$ years earlier.

Two patients suffered from a cardiac tumor. The first had an extensive fibroma involving the posterior wall of the right ventricle, the diaphragm, the upper part of the liver, and the left phrenic nerve satellite lymph nodes. The other patient had a carcinoma of the right heart involving the right atrium, the tricuspid valve, and the anterior wall of the inlet portion of the right ventricle.

Preoperative Condition

All patients but one were in functional Class III or IV before operation (Table 2). Nine patients had several episodes of pulmonary edema reversible

Table 2	
Patient Condition	
Functional Class (NYHA)	
Class III	10
Class IV	10
Associated Cardiac Lesions	
Mitral valve incompetence	2
Tricuspid valve incompetence	1
Associated Pathology	
Renal failure	8
Diabetes	7
Pulmonary hypertension	1
Obstructive pulmonary disease	3

under reinforced medical treatment, demonstrating a persistent "myocardial reserve." Eighteen patients were in sinus rhythm, but seven displayed ventricular extrasystoles among whom two had several episodes of ventricular tachycardia. Hemodynamic data and patients' condition are summarized in Table 3. The average ejection fraction in patients without left ventricular aneurysm ranged from 9% to 27% (mean 15.4%). Eight patients had renal failure, seven had diabetes, and three had chronic obstructive pulmonary disease.

Operation

With the exception of one patient who had a 4-week period of training of the latissimus dorsi muscle before the operation, all patients had a one-stage operation comprising latissimus dorsi dissection and transfer into the thorax with the patient in the lateral decubitus position and then a cardiomyoplasty with the patient in the dorsal decubitus position. In two patients who have been excluded from this series, a severe decrease in blood pressure when the patient was placed in lateral decubitus position before surgery led to cancellation of the operation because it was impossible to restore adequate blood pressure with cardiotonic drugs in this position. These two patients survived the anesthesia but died several months later. Of the 20 patients operated on, 13 benefited from the reinforcement technique, 5 from the substitution technique, and 2 from the combined substitution and reinforcement technique.

The postoperative follow-up of these patients is separated into two periods: a "preassist period" of 3 months—the time necessary to train the muscle and to reach its full power activity and an "assist period" beyond 3 months during which time the heart was effectively assisted by the muscle.

II. Preassist Period

The postoperative follow-up reflected the preoperative selection of the patients. Most patients had a difficult postoperative course. Only three remained in the ICU for less than 3 days and 11 for less than 6 days. Two patients remained in the ICU for 20 and 45 days, respectively.

Complications

Cardiac

Low cardiac output was the most frequent complication, presenting in six patients (30%). One patient died despite pharmacological support and two died despite associated mechanical support. In two patients, however, prolonged pharmacological support and mechanical support for 4 and 6 days, respectively were effective until the muscle could provide a valuable assistance (ninth week). Extrasystoles and episodes of ventricular fibrillation were present in one patient who eventually died.

Table 3

		Patient Condition					Operation				Follow-up	
No.	Pt.	Sex	Etiology	FC	Associated Lesions	EF (%)	Date	Type	Associated Treatment	ECC	Preassist P.	Late
01	PAS	F38	Tumor	IV	Liver extension Tamponade	45	Jan 85	S (Ant W)	Diaphragm resection Reconstruction	Yes	/	FC I
02	IOV	M59	Ischemic	IV	Diabetes LV aneurysm	12	Jul 85	S + R	Aneurysm	Yes	Death D3 LOW CO	/
03	FIL	M40	Ischemic	III	LV aneurysm	13	Apr 86	S + R	Resection aneurysm	No	Infection	FC II
04	ORT	M42	Ischemic	IV	Renal failure	13	May 86	R (Post W)	Resection aneurysm	No	Death D30 (Renal failure)	/
05	CER	M53	Ischemic	IV	/	10	Oct 86	R	/	No	/	Death 2 years (Infarct.)
06	FOR	M66	Ischemic	IV	Mitral insuf. Tricuspid insuf.	17	Jan 87	R	Mitral valvuloplasty Tricuspid valvuloplasty	Yes	Death D1 (Ventr. fib.)	/
07	HAM	M18	Cardiomyopathy	IV	Aort valve prost. Mitral repair	09	Mar 87	R	/	No	/	Death 2 years (Ventric. fib.)
08	GAV	M53	Cardiomyopathy	IV	Pulm. hypertens. Diabetes	11	Apr 87	R	Pierce Thoratec L + R assist	Yes	Death D1 (Ventr. fib.)	/
09	LED	M54	Ischemic	III	LV aneurysm	16	Jul 87	R + S	Resection aneurysm	Yes	/	FC II

No.	Name	Age/Sex	Etiology	FC	Associated	EF	Date	Technique	Procedure	ECC	Outcome	Result
10	REN	M52	Ischemic	IV	Diabetes Nephrectomy	16	Jul 87	R	Ant. descending bypass	Yes	Renal dial. Cholecyst.	FC II
11	LOR	M67	Ischemic	III	LV aneurysm Vent. tachycardia	23	Jul 87	R + S	Resection aneurysm	Yes	Death D2 (Low CO)	/
12	GAN	M55	Tumor	III	Tricuspid insuf.	35	Oct 87	S	Tricuspid bioprosthes. Right coro. bypass	Yes	Death D45 (Infection)	/
13	deB	M52	Ischemic	III	LV aneurysm	24	Apr 88	S + R	Resection aneurysm Marginal bypass	Yes	/	FC II
14	HAN	F56	Ischemic	III	Diabetes	16	Jul 88	S + R	Resection aneurysm Left marg. bypass	Yes	/	FC I
15	SEY	M50	Ischemic	III	/	10	Nov 88	R	/	No	/	FC II
16	PON	M61	Cardiomyopathy	IV	/	12	Dec 88	R	/	No	/	FC II
17	PER	M68	Cardiomyopathy	III	Pulm. hypertens. Diabetes	27	Feb 89	R	/	No	Death D66 (Respir. insuf.)	/
18	DEV	M47	Cardiomyopathy	III	Diabetes Hodgkin	27	Mar 89	R	/	No	/	FC II
19	PAS	M51	Cardiomyopathy	III	/	25	Jun 89	R	/	No	/	FC II
20	PEZ	M63	Ischemic	IV	LV aneurysm Diabetes	15	Jun 89	S + R	Resection aneurysm	Yes	/	FC II

FC = Functional Class (NYHA); EF = Ejection Fraction; S = Substitution technique; R = Reinforcement technique; ECC = Extracorporeal circulation.

Renal Failure

Renal failure seen in six patients (30%) was caused by poor preoperative condition, low cardiac output, and infection. Three patients had severe renal failure requiring renal dialysis. Two of them died. Three additional patients had creatinin augmentation. All patients were given dopamine 3 µg/kg/min in the days following operation.

Infection

Infection was present in 5 of 20 cases (25%). Two patients developed a general infection leading to death. In the three remaining cases, infection was localized to the area of dissection of the latissimus dorsi (2 cases) or to the pocket of the stimulator (1 case). The risk of infection was enhanced by the desperate condition of the patients selected, the length of the operation and the large area of dissection of the latissimus dorsi muscle.

Mortality (Table 4)

Seven patients (34%) died during the first 3-month period in spite of pharmacological support in all seven and mechanical support in three. Two of these seven patients died in the operating room from low cardiac output in spite of balloon counterpulsation or Pierce Thoratec ventricular assistance and pharmacological support. Two died from a low cardiac output in the first month following the operation. Two of these patients required renal dialysis because of associated renal failure. One patient who had episodes of ventricular tachycardia prior to the operation died from ventricular fibrillation. One patient died from renal failure and infection of the latissimus dorsi area of dissection 30 days after the operation, and one patient with a malignant tumor died 45 days after the operation from septicemia. With the exception of the patient

Table 4
Causes of Death

Preassist Period	*7/20 (35%)*
Low cardiac output	3
Ventricular fibrillation	2
Infection + tumor	1
Renal failure + infection	1
*Postassist Period**	*2/13 (15%)*
Arrhythmia	1
Myocardial infarction	1

* Follow-up: 3 months to 5 years (2.3 years)

Table 5
Preoperative Risk Factors and Mortality

	No. Patients	No. Deaths
Cardiac Function		
Functional Class IV	10	4
CO <3 L/min	6	4
Renal Failure	2	2
Pulmonary Hypertension	1	1
>50 mm Hg		
Obstructive Bronchitis	3	1

who died from infection of the latissimus dorsi area of dissection, these patients would have probably died within the same time frame without operation.

Risk Factors

The analysis of risk factors showed that ejection fraction, heart size, patient age, and cause of cardiac disease were not risk factors. The main risk factors were the functional class, the cardiac index, and associated pathologies. The number of deaths per number of patients at risk is indicated in Table 5. However, due to the small number of patients in this preliminary study definite conclusions cannot be established.

A better selection of patients, a systematic treatment of bronchitis as well as all potential sites of infection prior to the operation, and a significant reduction in the length of the operation have reduced the risk of this operation. There have been no hospital deaths in the last eight patients in our series.

III. Postassist Period

Thirteen patients have been followed for 3 months to 4.5 years postoperatively. The most striking feature in these patients has been functional improvement. All patients but one went from functional class III or IV to functional Class I, II, or III (Table 6). In most patients, improvement continued over a period of 6 months, but two patients experienced improvement up to 1 year. All patients but two patients returned to an almost normal social life.

One patient who improved from preoperative functional Class III to Class I displayed a sudden episode of heart failure with pulmonary edema 2 years postop. At admission, the Cardiomyostimulator™ Pulse Train Generator was found to be inoperative due to battery failure. It was immediately replaced by a new stimulator that provided a spectacular improvement of the patient's condition. Unfortunately, this patient died from arrhythmia some weeks later.

Table 6
Functional Improvement

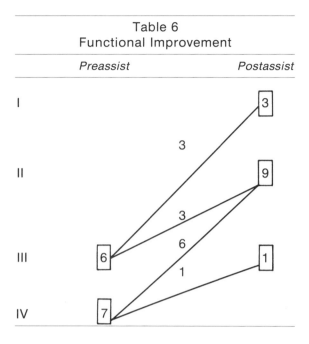

	Preassist	Postassist
I		3
II		9
III	6	1
IV	7	

Another patient died 2 years after the operation from recurrent myocardial infarction. Two patients required a cholecystectomy.

Hemodynamic Investigations

Cardiac Catheterization

Five of the 13 survivors agreed to be studied by cardiac catheterization more than 6 months postoperatively. The study was done after the full training of the latissimus dorsi (LD) had been completed. The following parameters were assessed: cardiac output by the Fick method, left ventricular diastolic pressures, and LV ejection fraction with the Cardio-Myostimulator™ IPG off and then with it on.

As an average, cardiac output increased from 4.2 L/min without stimulation to 51.1 L/min with stimulation, i.e. a 20% increase (Table 7). The most significant increase in CO was seen in a patient with a very low CO that rose from 3.3 L/min without stimulation to 6.3 L/min with stimulation.

Echo-Doppler Study

Two-dimensional and TM echocardiography and Doppler were carried out in the prestimulation period at each stage of the training period of the LD and

Table 7
Catheterization Results

Patient	CO		EF %		A/VD (vol%)	
	−	+	−	+	−	+
1	4.7	5.3	—	—	5.3	4.7
7	3.3	6.3	8	16	5.5	5.5
9	4.5	4.8	22	37	6.5	6
10	4	4.3	20	24	6.6	6
13	4.8	5.13	24	29	—	—

then every 6 months during the poststimulation period. Doppler study was done using a stand-alone Doppler system, Vingmed SD 100, which has the capability of automatic computation of the stroke volume and cardiac output. These parameters were studied as percentage variation in two clinical conditions: (a) burst stimulation of the LD 1:2 cardiac cycles and (b) without stimulation. Those two conditions were achieved during the same examination without any change of patient position or Doppler probe position. The aortic flow was interrogated by a 2.5 MHz probe in continuous wave emission. LV stroke volume was computed as the mean Y variation of the stimulated cycle against the nonstimulated cycle in a 1:2 stimulation program. The mean cardiac output per minute was expressed as a percentage variation between the basal condition without stimulation and the 1:2 cycle stimulation. Computing LV SV or CO by Doppler requires measurement of the aortic valve area in systole. This was estimated from the diameter of the aortic annulus assessed by 2D echocardiography. As the aortic area was kept as a constant in the various conditions in the same patients, the percentage variation of the SV and CO expressed the modification of the velocity time integral.

Nine patients were investigated at more than 6 months postoperatively (Table 8). Three of them did not show any modification of the LV ejection flow in the stimulated and nonstimulated cycles. Six had a 12% to 42% increase in stroke volume. In those six patients, CO increased from 7% to 19%.

Mugascan

99 MTC Scan was carried out at repeated intervals in six patients with a follow-up of more than 2 years. Table 9 shows an increase in ejection fraction similar to that found with other investigations. This increase remains the same between 1 year and 2 years postoperatively demonstrating the stability of the results.

Conclusions

From these results, several preliminary conclusions can be derived. The first is that continuous fatigueless muscular contraction under electrical stim-

Table 8
Echo-Doppler Studies
9 Patients >6 Months, Stimulation 1:2

Pt. No.	SV*	CO**
1	0	0
5	0	0
7	+42%	+19%
9	+12%	+7%
10	0	0
13	+23%	+10%
14	+18%	+13%
15	+29%	+11%
16	+10–50%	+0–18%

* % increase in stroke volume of the stimulated cycle compared to the nonstimulated cycle; ** % increase in CO under 1:2 stimulation compared to nonstimulated status.

Table 9
Hemodynamics Scan (Tc-99m) Ejection Fraction

Pt. No.	Preop	1987		1988	
		Off	On	Off	On
1	46	47	53	48	50
3	13	17	20	—	—
5	10	9	12	14	24
7	8	8	13	12	14
9	15	14	22	17	19.5
10	16	18	22	16	19
Average	12.4	13.2	17.8	14.7	19

ulation at the rate of the heart has been demonstrated for periods of more than 4 years. The second is that the management of these high risk patients during the preassist period is particularly demanding. The third is that all surviving patients were clinically improved and some displayed significant hemodynamic improvement. Hemodynamic improvement was moderate, however, and sometimes negligible making it difficult to explain the functional improvement. This is largely due to numerous technical factors that must be the object of future improvements.

References

1. Carpentier A, Chachques JC: Myocardial substitution with a stimulated skeletal muscle: first successful clinical case. Lancet 1:1267, 1985.
2. Carpentier A, Chachques JC: Latissimus dorsi cardiomyoplasty to increase cardiac output. In G Rabago, DA Cooley (eds): Heart Valve Replacement and Future Trends in Cardiac Surgery. Mount Kisco, NY, Futura Publishing Co, Inc, 1987, p 473.
3. Carpentier A, Chachques JC, Grandjean PA, et al: Dynamic cardiomyoplasty. Early clinical experience and preliminary conclusions. Proceedings 68th Annual Meeting of the American Association for Thoracic Surgery. Los Angeles, California, 1988, pp 64–65.
4. Chachques JC, Grandjean PA, Schwartz K, et al: Effect of latissimus dorsi dynamic cardiomyoplasty on ventricular function. Circulation 78 (Suppl 3):203, 1988.

Chapter 13

The Allegheny Hospital Experience

George J. Magovern, Ignacio Y. Christlieb, Race L. Kao*

To this day, very few aspects related to the clinical application of dynamic cardiomyoplasty are as challenging as the production of convincing, unequivocal data with which we can prove the beneficial effects this procedure has to offer those patients receiving it. For the last half decade, researchers from all disciplines involved with this intriguing capability of the striated muscle: namely to serve a function it was not created for, have been trying in vain to set a gold standard against which the efficiency of skeletal muscles to perform as a source of continuous mechanical energy can be measured.

Such function is now clinical reality in cases of dynamic cardiomyoplasty. At the time of the first international workshop in Paris, there were a total of 52 dynamic cardiomyoplasty cases reported by six different countries and eight separate surgical teams. In spite of enormous advances in medical technology for diagnosis and evaluation of literally every function in the human body, a test that can be used every time, display the highest degree of accuracy, and be reproducible and comparable has eluded everyone.

Cardiomyoplasty, by definition, is supposed to assist cardiac function and therefore improve that function. Thus, it is logical that only accepted procedures that test the heart for its properties are being used. It is for this reason that we judge the success or failure of a cardiomyoplasty procedure through such parameters as cardiac output, ejection fraction, stroke volume, peak pressure, contractility indices, end-diastolic volumes, etc.

We are focusing the best part of our clinical research on the follow-up of our patients. When evaluating patients during the postoperative period, we cannot help but ask if we are trying to judge a sick heart by what a muscular flap does for the heart or if are we trying to judge a skeletal muscle by how a sick heart responds to it. The answer is neither, because by wrapping the latissimus dorsi around the heart, we create a new entity, a binomial that is different from each part separately, and it should be considered, treated, and judged as such.

* With the cooperation of SB Park and GJ Magovern, Jr.
From *Cardiomyoplasty* edited by Alain Carpentier, MD, PhD, Juan-Carlos Chachques, MD, and Pierre Grandjean, MS © 1991. Futura Publishing Inc., Mount Kisco, NY.

Materials and Methods

Since September 9, 1985, seven patients have received a cardiomyoplasty at Allegheny General Hospital for conditions varying from left ventricular aneurysm to idiopathic dilated cardiomyopathy. Each one has been given essentially a different sensing/stimulating system. Four types of implantable pulse generators have been used in nine implants for six patients (Table 1). Patient 6 did not receive an IPG. The implant duration of one single IPG varied from 2 to 42 months, with an average of 14 months. Each patient also received a different set of leads. For the results to be understood, it is necessary to understand the different elements of the sensing/pacing systems used.

A bipolar sensing system, composed of two unipolar sutureless epicardial leads (Medtronic Model 4951) joined by a connecting lead adaptor kit (Medtronic Model 5866–24), was used in Case 1. Both electrodes were implanted in the right atrial wall. This was the only patient in our group in whom atrial sensing was used. An identical system was implanted for muscle stimulation, a proximal (−) electrode near the entry of the motor branch of the neurovascular pedicle and a distal (+) approximately 5 inches below near the midportion of the distal border. Both bipolar systems were connected to a Symbios™ dual-chamber pacemaker (Medtronic Model 7006).

A 4-lead as well was used in Case 2. Right ventricular sensing by an epicardial lead (Medtronic Model 4951) and a sutureless epicardial lead (Medtronic Model L917-T), connected to a Medtronic 5866–24 kit. A negative stimulating electrode (Medtronic Model 4951–35) was attached immediately adjacent to the main trunk of the thoracodorsal nerve at its entry point into the muscle. The positive electrode was a Medtronic Model 6917–53T lead in the

Table 1
Pulse Generators Implanted

Pt No.	Model	Duration	Problem
1	SYMBIOS 7006*	9/9/85–6/24/87	Insufficient Power
	DELTA 925†	6/24/87–2/10/89	Site Infection
2	SYMBIOS 7006	2/19/86–To Date	
3	ITREL 7420*	7/3/86–9/10/86	End of Service
	CMS—SP1005*	9/10/86–11/14/86	
4	DELTA 925†	2/11/87–3/23/89	End of Life
	DELTA 925†	3/23/89–To Date	
5	DELTA 925†	9/7/88–To Date	
6	–	–	
7	CMS—SP1005*	3/23/89–To Date	

CMS = Cardiomyostimulator™; * Medtronic Inc., Minneapolis, MN; † Cardiac Pacemakers, Inc., (CPI) at St. Paul, MN.

insulation of six 1-mm^2 windows that had been opened to stimulate a wider spread of muscular fibers. A Medtronic Model 5866–24 connector was used. Both bipolar ends were connected to a Symbios™ 7006 (Medtronic).

The same muscular pacing leads arrangement connected during a first operation to an Itrel™ neurostimulator (Medtronic Model 7420) was implanted in Case 3. The latissimus dorsi muscle was stimulated for a period of 10 weeks to convert the fibers to a fatigue-resistant type. When cardiac surgery was performed, an epicardial sensing lead, Sentra Model 4315 (CPI) was implanted in the right ventricular wall. This and the pacing leads were connected 3 weeks later with a 5866–24 Medtronic connector to an SP1005 Cardiomyostimulator™ Pulse Train Generator. Stimulation started after a 10-day obligatory "resting" period using the secong phase of the program of stimulation to accelerate the training process.

Case 4 received a sutureless myocardial lead (CPI Model 4312) implanted with 1½ loops around the thoracodorsal nerve. Care was taken to avoid trauma and to fix the head of the lead to the surrounding muscular fibers. The anodic (+) Medtronic Model 6917–53T lead was modified in the same manner as in cases 2 and 3. A lead adapter (CPI Model 6021) was used to join the bipolar system. A Sentra Model 4315 unipolar lead was implanted in the right ventricular wall for sensing. Both pins were connected to a dual-chamber pulse generator Delta™-type Model 925 (CPI).

Case No. 5 was given a Medtronic Model 4315 sensing lead and a modified CPI Sentra Model 4260 bipolar endocardial porous tined tip for pacing. Both distal and proximal electrodes of this lead were previously shielded towards the "back" of the lead with ⅜-inch diameter pieces of reinforced silastic sheet 0.02 inches thick and fixed to the lead with 5–0 blue monofilament polypropylene surgical suture. Both "low profile" connecting pins were attached to a Delta™ 925 (CPI) programmed accordingly.

Case 6 received three pacing leads (Medtronic Model SP5528). The pair of leads that elicited the best contraction was connected by a Medtronic Model 5866–24 connector, and a low-profile sensing lead Medtronic Model 4315 was implanted in the right ventricular wall. Both pins were pulled through a tunnel into a subcutaneous pouch in the left hypochondrium where a stimulator was to be implanted. Due to postoperative complications, however, the stimulator was not implanted.

Case 7 received two Medtronic Model SP5528 leads in the proximal portion of the latissimus dorsi. When tested, an excellent muscular contraction was elicited. The patient also received a Medtronic Model 4313 lead for right ventricular sensing. These were connected to the muscular and cardiac ports of a Cardiomyostimulator™ Pulse Train Generator (Medtronic Model SP1005), which was turned "ON" on the 10th postoperative day to begin muscular fiber transformation.

We have followed a very similar latissimus dorsi muscle flap "conditioning" protocol in all of our patients. Based on our animal experience, we are convinced that it is safer to provide long resting periods at the beginning of the transforming period and gradually increase the stimulator output and "working" time to reach optimal electric energy delivery and 24 hours continuous pacing at the end of 6 weeks. The basic calendar distribution of this protocol consists of 2 × 2 hours the first week, 4 × 2 hours the second, 8 hours continuously the third week, 12 hours, 10 hours, and 24 hours continuously the fourth, fifth, and sixth weeks, respectively. Energy output should be gauged by the reaction of the individual patient. For more details on the surgical procedures for these patients the reader is referred to Chapter 11.

Results

To attempt statistical analysis of the results obtained in this reduced group of patients would be unrealistic. The one parameter that measures the degree of performance of the heart-muscle binomial: the cardiomyoplasty or cardiomyopexy entity and succeeds in achieving a fair comparison between the stimulated and the nonstimulated modes has not been established. Until that parameter is established, the best option is to select the noninvasive tests of choice and use them, everything else being the same, with the muscle flap in the two controlled situations. Since invasive procedures rarely are accepted by patients today, we have used M-mode, two-dimensional, and Doppler echocardiography and exercise multiple gated acquisition (MUGA) studies after injection of a titrated dose of Tc-99m pertechnetate. The basic requested information has been wall motion, cardiac output, and ejection fraction.

The following is a discussion of Case 1, MJ, who in 1989 was 45 months postsurgery.[1,2] Her first pacemaker, implanted subcutaneously in the left hypochondrium, started to erode through the skin as early as three weeks postimplant (PI) but healed before discharge from the hospital. At 14 months PI her IPG was surgically relocated to a deeper pouch because of erosion. At 21 months PI this pacer became asynchronous and could not be converted to synchrony under any available program. A decision was made to replace it with another model with a broader programming capability (Table 1), which restored synchrony. By this time, the patient had moved from Pennsylvania to Louisiana. She returned 3 weeks later because of erosion of the lead wires through the skin. Lead wires were repositioned to a deeper layer. Two months later a fourth readmission was necessary for treatment of the same condition. This time the lead wires were transposed to under the rectus fascia and muscle fibers. Six months later a 1-cm diameter area of superficial erosion without local reaction was noted. The patient was instructed to keep the area clean and antibiotics were prescribed. Six months later she returned with severe inflammatory reaction over the pacemaker site and the dual-barrel connectors and an open infected wound below the xyphoid, through which all four lead wires were showing. Once again, extensive debridement of the area and repositioning of the exposed lead sections was carried out under heavy antibiotic therapy. Five months later (40 months PI), the pacemaker was explanted in an attempt to facilitate the treatment by reducing the amount of foreign material in the area. On February 10, 1989, she was taken to the operating room, and the surface area of the left ventricular wall was estimated both in systole and diastole through a short-axis echocardiographic view. Cardiac outputs

Table 2
Echocardiography—Short-Axis L.V. case 1 2/10/89

	Syst. S.A.[a]	Diast S.A.[b]	% Change[c]
Old Pacemaker*	13.4 cm²	24.2 cm²	45
Fresh Pacemaker	12.6 cm²	24.4 cm²	48
No Stimulator	9.7 cm²	16.7 cm²	42
Burst Stimulator 1:1	8.6 cm²	19.3 cm²	56
Burst Stimulator 2:1	9.6 cm²	23.8 cm²	60

S.A. = Surface area; * Prior to pacemaker manipulation; [a] Normal range 4.0–11.6 cm²; [b] Normal range 9.5–22.3 cm²; [c] Normal range 36%–64%.

were measured by the thermodilution technique. The same measurements were repeated with a new pacemaker of the same model (Delta™ 925, CPI) with the flap not being stimulated and with 1:1 and 2:1 burst stimulation using a Cardiomyostimulator™ Pulse Train Generator (Medtronic SP1005). The results are shown in Table 2. Cardiac outputs determined while testing these different pacing modes revealed a 1,000 mL difference between the flap not being stimulated (4,000 mL/min) and burst stimulation (5,000 mL/min). The two single stimulus devices fell in between: 4,200 mL/min for the worn out Delta™ 925 stimulator and 4,700 mL/min for the fresh one.

Prior to this point, cardiac outputs as calculated by Doppler echocardiography, had been improving for the previous 2 years with and without stimulation, but the difference between the two modes was not significant (Fig 1). Her progress through 3 ½ years as evaluated by left ventricular ejection fraction is shown in Figure 2. These values are from stress MUGA studies at 50-watt level of exercise. It should be noted that the peak benefit from her operation appears to have been reached during the second year after surgery. At this time, the "dynamic" part of her cardiomyoplasty is on hold. The persistence of infection made it necessary to eliminate the two dual-barrel lead adaptors and eventually the connecting pin ends of all four leads. She remains in the follow-up program.

In 1989 Case 2, JR, was 42 months postcardiomyoplasty.[3] Although his improvement by all subjective parameters has been outstanding, his LVEF never showed any significant difference, particularly during exercise (Fig 3). During the second year postsurgery the benefit appeared to be the best. Resting cardiac output improved with stimulation up to 2½ years PI (Fig. 4), but this did not last. The patient was due for pacer replacement and theoretically a new device should result in some improvement.

Case 3, RW, received a Cardiomyostimulator™ Pulse Train Generator (Medtronic Model SP1005 after the latissimus was preconditioned with an Itrel™ (Medtronic Model 7420). He expired the day he was being discharged (2 months after surgery), most likely from a fatal arrhythmia. Autopsy revealed an infected and degenerated muscle flap and a fractured proximal pacing lead (Medtronic Model 4951). His case has been described elsewhere.[3]

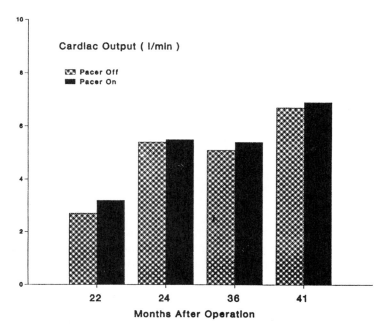

Figure 1. *Cardiac output as determined by Doppler echocardiography on patient MJ, Case 1, at two years and up to the time of pacer removal.*

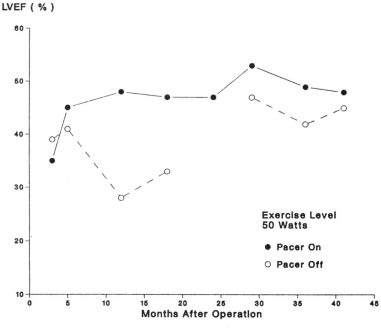

Figure 2. *Case 1, MJ, from surgery to pacer removal. Left ventricular ejection fraction (%) as determined by MUGA scan during exercise. Report is at a level of 50 watts. At the 24–month study, the patient did not reach this level with the pacer OFF.*

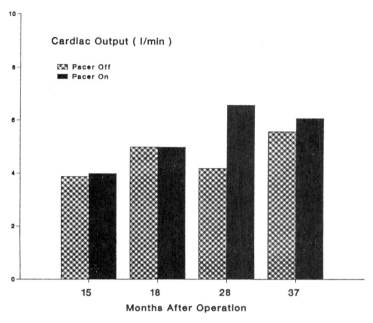

Figure 3. *Case 2, JR, from surgery to the last study at 37 months. Left ventricular ejection fraction (LVEF) (%) as determined by MUGA scan during exercise. Report is at a level of 75 watts. Peak performance shows at 15 months.*

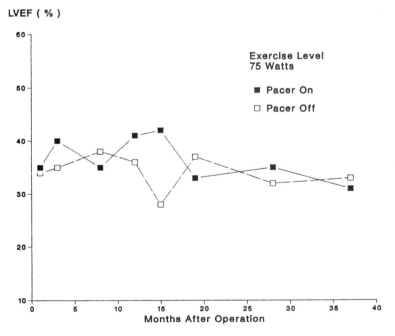

Figure 4. *Case 2, JR, cardiac output as determined by Doppler echocardiography during second and third postoperative years. Peak performance shows at 28 months while there is no difference at 15 months. Follow-up at 37 months suggests low IPG battery or need for an IPG with higher electrical output.*

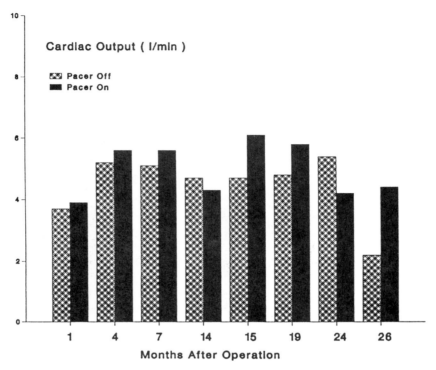

Figure 5. *Case 4, MM, from surgery to the last study at 26 months after IPG replacement. Peak performance shows during second year at 15 and 19 months. Asynchronous pacing (VVI) at 24 months required immediate replacement. The patient in mild CHF at the time of this test.*

Case 4, MM, was a 67-year-old female, who in 1989 was 28 months PI and in the third month of her second IPG. She was a Class IV patient, but was reclassified to Class III-IV. She was limited by severe arteriosclerosis, diabetes mellitus, and arterial hypertension. Her clinical progress was remarkable inasmuch as she was in severe refractory cardiac failure before surgery, in need of hospitalization at least 50% of the time, and totally unresponsive to medical therapy. Since surgery she has been hospitalized only a few times, at first because of chronic heart failure caused by her falling in atrial fibrillation, the flap becoming asynchronous with the ventricles, and more recently, because her stimulator reached end-of-life period, which caused asynchrony (solved by stimulator replacement) and because of severe lower limb claudication that required laser angioplasty. This case also illustrates the maximum benefit of the procedure during the second postoperative year (Fig. 5) and the dramatic effect of replacing a rundown battery (24 months) with a new one (26 months). The patient returned to normal activity with no additional medical problems.

Case 5, BD, was only 9 months postsurgery in 1989, and her initial studies, at 1½ and 6 months PI are totally unrevealing (Table 3). She was a 65-year-old female, who was a diabetic and a hypertensive, spending 50% of her time

Table 3
Left Ventricular Ejection Fraction—Case 5

	Echo		Rest MUGA	
Pacer:	OFF	ON	OFF	ON
Preop	32%		24%	
1.5 Mo Postop	36%	38%	26%	28%
6 Mo Postop	36%	38%	30%	33%

in a hospital to be diuresed and barely improved from uncontrollable chronic heart failure. She had not had a single admission since her cardiomyoplasty.

Case 6, RM, was a 61-year-old transplant candidate who choose not to consider the option of heart transplantation. He had an extremely severe ischemic cardiomyopathy in chronic heart failure, with a left ventricular ejection fraction (EF) of 14% and a 15% EF at rest in the right ventricle. Since there was an aneurysmal sac in the left ventricular wall and there was a possibility of resection and/or a coronary artery bypass graft, he was placed on cardiopulmonary bypass for the cardiac stage of the procedure. During that procedure, a large amount of blood accumulated at the latissimus dorsi muscle dissection site that rendered the patient hypovolemic and acutely anemic. Multiple blood and blood products were transfused and reoperation was necessary. Severe hemodilution developed and multiple-organ failure ensued, which eventually caused his death four weeks after the operation, without ever having had a stimulator implanted.

Case 7, RB, was a 59-year-old male with idiopathic dilated cardiomyopathy 2½ months postsurgery on whom the cardiomyoplasty was staged allowing 48 hours between the freeing of the latissimus dorsi and its wrapping around the heart. This, plus the fact that cardiopulmonary bypass was not used, are probably the two most decisively determining factors for his quick and uncomplicated recovery. Table 4 depicts the results of his echocardiographic and MUGA studies at 1, 1½, and 2 months postsurgery. It should be noted that after the first month, at which time he was only 2 weeks into the fiber transformation period, the results seem paradoxical in that the stroke volume of the nonpaced beats, thus the resultant cardiac output, are higher than those of the paced beats. Furthermore, stroke volume and cardiac output when the pacer is turned OFF are significantly higher than when turned ON.

Discussion

Cardiomyoplasty is still a young procedure, the first case having been performed in 1985.[4] There is still much to be learned. The accumulated experience in follow-up and late results is limited. There is little comparative data available in the literature[3,5–7] and there is a painful lack of standard

Table 4
Left Ventricular Ejection Fraction—Case 7

	Echo		Rest MUGA	
Pacer:	OFF	ON	OFF	ON
Preop	16%		22%	
1 Mo Postop	23%	27%	18%	20%

Doppler Echocardiography—Case 7

	LV Stroke VOL (mL/beat)				Cardiac Output (L/min)			
		ON				ON		
Pacer:	OFF	NPB	PB	Avg	OFF	NPB	PB	Avg
1.5 Mo Postop	56	47	43	45	4.8	4.6	4.2	4.4
2 Mo Postop	56	55	38	46.5	4.4	4.8	2.6	3.7

NPB = Nonpaced beat; PB = Paced beat.

tests for evaluation of the procedure. In addition, there are an immense number of variables within the surgical technique, which makes grouping the cases, even within a single surgical group, an almost impossible task.

The purpose in writing this chapter was to provide an analysis of our practice of nearly four years, to recognize our attainments as well as our flaws, and to benefit from our own experience as well as from that of others in the field. Five out of seven of our patients survived the operation and have a better quality of life than before surgery. Four have survived and claimed improvement on DDD pacemakers and adapted cardiac pacing leads. One patient died at 1 month and another at 2 months postoperatively. They were transplant candidates who had refused the idea of accepting a donor's heart. Both patients were accepted for a burst pacemaker protocol because of their poor condition, but died before receiving the benefit of biomechanical cardiac assistance.

An analysis of the results presented here is mostly an analysis of the use of DDD pulse generators in the cardiomyoplasty procedure. Not enough data is yet available regarding the only burst generator (Medtronic Model SP1005). However, there is evidence at 2 months (Table 4) that while cardiac output is higher with the pacer OFF, cardiac rate increases 45% and systolic pressure decreases 6%, with the pacer ON at the same exercise level, heart rates increases 41% and systolic blood pressure increases by 20%. This was coincident with the end of the fiber transformation period and could be due, next to the important role played by the systemic peripheral resistances, to the fact that a larger percentage of muscular fibers are now "slow," type I, and therefore have lost some power. This would indicate a need for adjustments in the pacing program.

Thus far it has been proven that it is possible to transform muscular fibers with a single pulse stimulator as well as with burst stimulation. We are now studying a series of patients on whom permanent stimulation will be of the burst type. Permanent programs will be studied one at a time and readjusted according to the results of each test.

This brings us back to the subject of "the test." Our early experience with single pulse stimulators has been evaluated by echocardiographic and MUGA studies translated into ejection fraction and/or cardiac output. Experiences with patients 1, 2, and 4 suggest that flap performance reaches a peak during the course of the second year after the operation and that the differential gap between function with the flap ON and the flap OFF begins to narrow again after that point. Our studies indicate that when the pulse generator is replaced (Table 2, Fig. 5), the differential gap opens up again, but narrows still more (Figs. 3 and 4) if the pulse generator is not replaced. The accuracy of this hypothesis will be determined when Case 2 is tested after IPG replacement.

Perhaps the end-of-life point in an active pulse generator as we know it is not good enough when programmed to the kind of energy settings needed to stimulate a skeletal muscle as opposed to those in pacing a heart. Perhaps the "prophylactic" replacement at 21 months, as specified by the FDA-Medtronic-AGH protocol for the SP1005, is not that much of a waste in battery energy of an otherwise perfectly good device as it appears to be to some of us. Prophylactic replacement should not only be accepted, but perhaps enthusiastically endorsed.

Our transient experience with a burst stimulator on a skeletal muscle flap otherwise stimulated to contract for more than 3 years (Table 2) may shed some light on future considerations for SP1005 use. Contraction goes up with burst stimulation Mode I and II. Single pulse stimulation does not seem to affect this parameter. Relaxation is essentially the same whether there is no stimulation, a good single-pulse pacemaker, or a 2:1 program (Mode II) with a burst stimulator. This stresses the importance of providing for good diastolic filling, particularly of the right ventricular cavity, at surgery and when programming the stimulator, and consideration to the intrinsic heart rate, if one is to maintain good cardiac output.

The quest continues for a working, permanent, long-term left ventricular dysfunction experimental model that will investigate and find that "gold standard" for testing cardiomyoplasty procedures for functional adequacy.

It is unfortunate that in all of our hospital survivors, the patient's own subjective feeling of improvement, dramatic as it may be at times, cannot be matched by any single test of "cardiac" performance as we know them today and that these so-called testimonial arguments are condemned to remain invalid for lack of measurable parameters amenable to statistical analysis.

References

1. Magovern GJ, Park SB, Magovern GJ Jr., et al: Latissimus dorsi as a functioning synchronously paced muscle component in the repair of a left ventricular aneurysm. Ann Thorac Surg 41:116, 1986.

2. Magovern GJ, Heckler FR, Park SB, et al: Paced latissimus dorsi used for dynamic cardiomyoplasty of left ventricular aneurysms. Ann Thorac Surg 44:379, 1987.
3. Magovern GJ, Heckler FR, Park SB, et al: Paced skeletal muscle for dynamic cardiomyoplasty. Ann Thorac Surg 45:614, 1988.
4. Carpentier A, Chachques JC: Myocardial substitution with a stimulated skeletal muscle: first successful clinical case. Lancet i:1267, 1985.
5. Carpentier A, Chachques JC: Latissimus dorsi cardiomyoplasty to increase cardiac output. Clinical experience. In G Rabago, D Cooley (eds): Heart Valve Replacement: Current Status and Future Trends. Mount Kisco, NY, Futura Publishing Co, 1987, pp 473–486.
6. Chachques JC, Grandjean MS, Schwartz K, et al: Effect of latissimus dorsi dynamic cardiomyoplasty on ventricular function. Circulation 78:III-203, 1988.
7. Molteni L, Almada H, Ferreira R: Synchronously stimulated skeletal muscle graft for left ventricular assistance. J Thorac Cardiovasc Surg 97:439, 1989.

Chapter 14

Cardiomyoplasty in Dilated Cardiomyopathy

Luiz Felipe P. Moreira, Adib D. Jatene*

Initially described by Carpentier and Chachques in 1985,[1] cardiomyoplasty has been proposed as a myocardial substitute in the treatment of left ventricular tumors or aneurysms[2-5] and as a method of biomechanical ventricular assistance in patients with dilated or ischemic cardiomyopathy.[2,6,7]

Experimental reports showed that skeletal muscles are capable of performing hemodynamic work with the use of pulse train electrical stimulation[8-10] and that sustained work without fatigue is possible after a period of continuous electrical conditioning.[11-13] In addition, some authors described the maintenance of normal cardiac output when right or left ventricular walls were partially replaced by synchronous stimulated skeletal muscles.[3,14] Our group also demonstrated the improvement of left ventricular performance with a muscle flap wrapped around the ventricular walls that contracted synchronously with the heart in the presence of acutely induced myocardial dysfunction.[15,16]

Thus far, clinical experience with cardiomyoplasty includes only a limited number of cases[1-7] in heterogeneous groups of patients and with sometimes inadequate muscle stimulation devices.[4,5,7]

However, this surgical procedure seems to have less important mortality when it is performed without the use of cardiopulmonary bypass, which is only mandatory in the presence of associated procedures such as the resection of left ventricular tumors or aneurysms, myocardial revascularization, and valvular reconstruction or replacement.[2] In this chapter, we would like to discuss the use of cardiomyoplasty in dilated cardiomyopathy.

Despite the promising results of cardiac transplantation,[17] this procedure does have limitations, including restricted availability of donor organs and the adverse effects of immunosuppressive therapy.[18] As a result, dilated cardiomyopathy, which is present in more than 50% of transplantation candidates,[17] remains a significant cause of death, especially in South America where there is a high incidence of Chagas' disease.[19]

---

* With the cooperation of NAG Stolf, EA Bocchi, and AC Pereira-Barreto.

From *Cardiomyoplasty* edited by Alain Carpentier, MD, PhD, Juan-Carlos Chachques, MD, and Pierre Grandjean, MS © 1991. Futura Publishing Inc., Mount Kisco, NY.

	Mean	SD
Table 1 Preoperative Data		
Cardiothoracic index	58	3%
Left ventricular diastolic diameter (Echo)	75	11 mm
Left ventricular ejection fraction (MUGA)	21	5%
Cardiac index (Thermodilution)	1.7	0.3 L/min.m²
Left ventricular end-diastolic pressure	26	7 mm Hg
Presence of mitral regurgitation	6 patients	

Clinical Protocol

From May 1988 to May 1989, eight patients with dilated cardiomyopathy and medical or psychosocial contraindications to cardiac transplantation were presented for cardiomyoplasty at the Sao Paulo Heart Institute. Etiology was idiopathic in six patients and Chagas' disease in two patients. All patients were male and age ranged from 16 to 53 years. At the time of the operation, five patients were in NYHA Class III and three in Class IV, despite maximal medical therapy. One patient presented chronic atrial fibrillation, and five had nonsustained ventricular tachycardia episodes on Holter monitor recordings. The morphological and hemodynamic characteristics of the patients' heart are presented in Table 1.

Surgical Procedure

Cardiomyoplasty was performed using the reinforcement technique described by Carpentier and Chachques[2] without the use of cardiopulmonary bypass. The left latissimus dorsi muscle was dissected through a lateral incision preserving the neurovascular pedicle. The muscle flap was transposed into the left hemithorax through a window created by partial resection of the second rib. A longitudinal sternotomy was then performed, the heart exposed by a wide opening of the pericardium, and the muscle flap wrapped around the left and right ventricles with its paravertebral and superior edges fixed along the posterior atrioventricular line. The previously implanted intramuscular electrodes (Medtronic Model SP5528 BV) and the epicardial sensing lead (Medtronic Model SP5548 BV) were connected to the Cardiomyostimulator™ Pulse Train Generator (Medtronic SP1005 BV) located in the abdominal wall. The left latissimus dorsi muscle wrapped more than 85% of the left ventricular wall in all procedures and more than 50% of the right ventricular wall.

There were no operative deaths, and the prophylactic use of sympathomimetic amines and vasodilators provided an adequate hemodynamic condition during the surgical procedure and the immediate postoperative period in every patient. However, a transitory period of renal failure and mesenteric ischemia was observed during the first week after the operation in the fifth patient. This was associated with an important increase of the plasmatic creatinophosphokinase enzyme level on the third postoperative day.

The muscle stimulation protocol was started 2 weeks after cardiomyoplasty. At that time, the patient who had enzymatic alterations in the immediate postoperative period presented absence of muscle flap contraction with maximal electrical stimulation. This patient died 2 months later in congestive heart failure; latissimus dorsi normal fibers intermediated by areas of fibrosis were documented by microscopic study. The other seven patients followed the progressive stimulation protocol proposed by Carpentier and Chachques[2,3] with normal response.

Clinical and Hemodynamic Evaluation

Two patients remained in the course of muscle stimulation protocol at the time of this publication and were in NYHA Class II under medical therapy. The other five patients completed the muscle conditioning period and were followed from 6 to 14 months. Three patients were in NYHA Class I and returned to their professional activities, one patient was in Class II and another in Class III, some of them using lesser amounts of drugs in comparison to the preoperative period.

Laboratory investigation was undertaken in the third and sixth postoperative months to evaluate the functional and hemodynamic influence of cardiomyoplasty. Figure 1 shows the results of maximal oxygen consumption during a treadmill test using the Naughton protocol. The significant difference of the data obtained before and after the operation ($+52\% \pm 8\%$) confirmed the better exercise tolerance of the patients in the postoperative period.

The left ventricular function changes after cardiomyoplasty were documented by echocardiographic study (Table 2) and by Technetium pool-gated ventriculography (Fig. 2). These studies showed an important improvement of the left ventricular wall shortening ($+53\% \pm 10\%$) and ejection fraction ($+31\% \pm 7\%$), as exemplified in Figure 3. In addition, a better hemodynamic condition was also observed at rest by cardiac catheterization and the thermodilution method (Table 3). However, it is important to emphasize that the patients who had greater left ventricular dimensions presented a less evident variation of left ventricular function.

Furthermore, it was also possible to document the reduction of ventricular tachyarrhythmias in four of the five patients that completed the muscle conditioning period on Holter monitor recordings without the use of specific medical therapy (Fig. 4).

Finally, the evaluation of the pulmonary function showed that the presence of the latissimus dorsi muscle in the left hemithorax lead to a vital capacity decrease of $18.4\% \pm 2.3\%$ ($p < 0.04$). Nevertheless, this finding was not responsible for any clinical symptomatology.

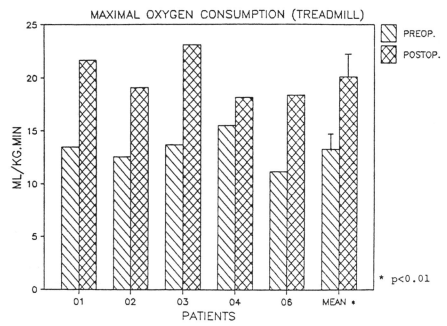

Figure 1. *Maximal oxygen consumption during treadmill tests performed before and after cardiomyoplasty.*

Table 2
Echocardiographic Evaluation of the Left Ventricular Function

	Diastolic Diameter (mm)		Wall Shortening (%)	
	Preop.	*Postop.*	*Preop.*	*Postop.*
Case 1	62	65	12	20
Case 2	64	70	16	20
Case 3	74	75	15	21
Case 4	89	86	7	13
Case 6	82	82	8	12
Mean ± SD	74 ± 11	75 ± 8	11 ± 4	17 ± 4
	Not Significant		$p < 0.01$	

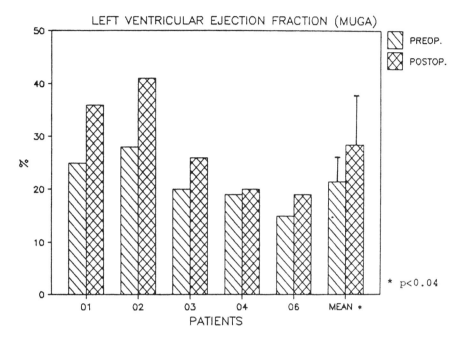

Figure 2. *Left ventricular ejection fraction determinations by multiple-gated angiography (MUGA) in the pre- and postoperative periods.*

Table 3
Hemodynamic Evaluation of the Left Ventricular Function

	Stroke Work Index (gr.m/m2)		Pulm Wedge Pressure (mm Hg)	
	Preop.	*Postop.*	*Preop.*	*Postop.*
Case 1	18.7	27	16	5
Case 2	10.1	16.3	25	22
Case 3	14.7	26.3	30	13
Case 4	18.3	21.6	23	21
Case 6	9.2	16.2	30	25
Mean ± SD	14.1 ± 4.4	21.5 ± 5.2	25 ± 6	17 ± 8
	$p < 0.01$		$p < 0.04$	

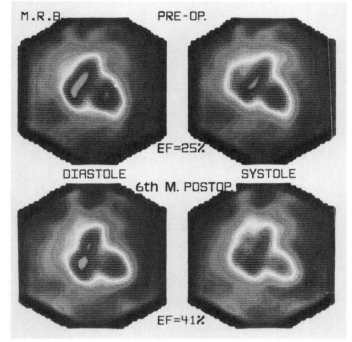

Figure 3. *Left ventricular multiple-gated angiographies obtained in the preoperative period and 6 months after cardiomyoplasty.*

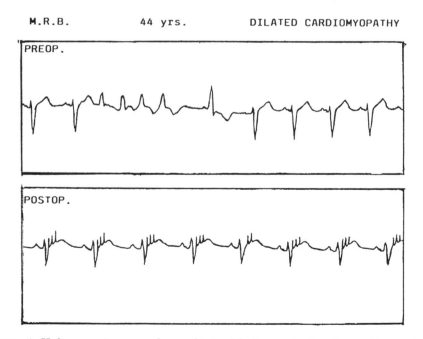

Figure 4. *Holter monitor recordings obtained before and after the cardiomyoplasty.*

Discussion

Cardiomyoplasty in the treatment of dilated cardiomyopathy aims to improve the patient's functional capacity and slow the evolution of the disease as a result of better performance of the reinforced ventricles.

In the initial clinical experience with this new surgical technique, the selection of patients followed the same criteria currently used for cardiac transplantation.[3,21] Only patients identified as being at risk of dying from myocardial dysfunction were considered candidates for the procedure. However, it is important to emphasize that cardiomyoplasty requires a delay of 2 weeks to start latissimus dorsi muscle stimulation. This time period is necessary to provide an adequate adhesion between the muscle fibers and neighboring structures[2,4] and muscle flap vascular adaptation.[22] This fact may represent a limitation for the indication of this operation in patients with end-stage cardiac failure shock.

Furthermore, the existence of severe mitral regurgitation and important enlargement of the left ventricle, which occurs in a high percentage of patients with dilated cardiomyopathy,[19,23,24] also has been suggested to represent a contraindication for cardiomyoplasty[3,25] In the present investigation, the occurrence of a less important improvement of the ventricular function in a patient with greater left ventricular dimensions justifies this proposition and suggests that the indications for cardiomyoplasty need to be defined differently than for heart transplantation.

A low immediate mortality rate, as documented by the present data and other authors can be achieved when this operation is performed without the use of cardiopulmonary bypass.[2,6,7] Adequate management of the patients' circulatory condition during the surgical procedure and the postoperative period plays also an important role in the success of the operation, providing a low complication rate and a more uneventful recovery. The present experience emphasizes the value of the prophylactic use of drugs to maintain normal cardiac performance in patients after this surgical injury, including patients with severe myocardial dysfunction. The availability of mechanical circulatory assist devices is also important.

The maintenance of a stable circulatory condition also plays an important role in preventing muscle flap ischemia. The occurrence of muscle flap damage with loss of skeletal muscle response to electrical stimulation has been reported in an experimental study[26] and was observed in one patient in this investigation. The adequate preservation of latissimus dorsi vascular supply during cardiomyoplasty and of normal muscle perfusion in the immediate postoperative period minimizes the risk of this complication that can be identified by the monitoring of creatinophosphokinase enzyme variation.

Pulmonary dysfunction represents another limitation for the utilization of this technique. In spite of the absence of any clinical symptomatology due to this alteration in our experience, patients with previous pulmonary diseases are not recommended as candidates for cardiomyoplasty.

Parallel to previous reports that demonstrated improvement of ventricular function due to cardiomyoplasty in patients with left ventricular tumors or aneurysms[2,4,5] and with cardiomyopathies,[2,5–7] our initial clinical experience with this technique in the treatment of dilated cardiomyopathy showed significant changes in cardiac performance. An important increment in left ventricular ejection fraction was observed after the operation and occurred with the maintenance of the same left ventricular dimensions. This fact was responsible for a significant stroke work index augmentation and an important decrease in the pulmonary wedge pressure.

Furthermore, the improvement of the hemodynamic status due to cardiomyoplasty provided a better clinical condition and an increase in patients' exercise performance, documented by maximal oxygen consumption monitoring during treadmill testing. It is important to emphasize that in some patients these results were obtained with the use of lesser amounts of drugs than were used in the preoperative period. As suggested previously,[25] this better control of the congestive failure state may improve life expectancy with dilated cardiomyopathy, a concept corroborated by the maintenance of cardiomyoplasty benefits for more than one year in some of our patients. The hemodynamic improvement with this technique results in a better myocardial contraction efficiency due to cardiac performance augmentation without the participation of the myocardial fibers. This may explain the reduction of ventricular tachyarrhythmias we have observed in our experience.

Conclusion

Our limited experience confirms that cardiomyoplasty may be performed without the use of cardiopulmonary bypass in patients with dilated cardiomyopathy with an acceptable immediate mortality. The surgical morbidity of this procedures appears to be limited to the possibility of muscle flap damage and pulmonary function impairment resulting from the muscular mass within the left pleural cavity. Cardiomyoplasty may increase ventricular contractility, provide better control of congestive heart failure, and improve the functional determinants of survival in the treatment of dilated cardiomyopathy.

The benefits of this new surgical technique seems to be better in patients with only moderate increase of ventricular dimensions. The indications for this operation need to be defined on the basis of a larger experience and on criteria that are different than that of cardiac transplantation.

References

1. Carpentier A, Chachques JC: Myocardial substitution with a stimulated skeletal muscle: first successful clinical case (letter). Lancet 8440:1267, 1985.
2. Carpentier A, Chachques JC, Grandjean P, et al: dynamic Cardiomyoplasty. Early clinical experience and preliminary conclusions. Proceedings of the 68th Annual Meeting of the American Association for Thoracic Surgery, Los Angeles, U.S.A., 1988, pp 64–65.
3. Chachques JC, Grandjean P, Schwartz K, et al: Effect of latissimus dorsi dynamic cardiomyoplasty on ventricular function. Circulation 78(suppl. 3):203, 1988.

4. Magovern GJ, Heckler FR, Park SB, et al: Paced latissimus dorsi used for dynamic cardiomyoplasty of left ventricular aneurysms. Ann Thorac Surg 44:379, 1987.
5. Magovern GJ, Heckler FR, Park SB, et al: Paced skeletal muscle for dynamic cardiomyoplasty. Ann Thorac Surg 45:614, 1988.
6. Dumcius A, Salcius K, Giedraits S, et al: Myoventriculoplasty with the use of programmed physiologically controlled electroneurostimulation (letter). J Thorac Cardiovasc Surg 97:636, 1989.
7. Molteni L, Almada H, Ferreira R: Synchronously stimulated skeletal muscle graft for left ventricular assistance. J Thorac Cardiovasc Surg 97:439, 1989.
8. Acker MA, Anderson WA, Hammond RL, et al: Skeletal muscle ventricles in circulation. One to eleven weeks' experience. J Thorac Cardiovasc Surg 94:613, 1987.
9. Chiu RC-J, Walsh GL, Dewar ML, et al: Implantable extra-aortic balloon assist powered by transformed fatigue-resistant skeletal muscle. J Thorac Cardiovasc Surg 94:694, 1987.
10. Mannion JD, Acker MA, Hammond RL, et al: Power output of skeletal muscle ventricles in circulation: short-term studies. Circulation 76:155, 1987.
11. Leirner A, Moreira LFP, Chagas ACP, et al: Biomechanical circulatory assistance. Importance of aerobic capacity of normal and conditioned skeletal muscles. Trans Am Soc Artif Intern Organs 34:716, 1988.
12. Mannion JD, Bitto T, Hammond RL, et al: Histochemical and fatigue characteristics of conditioned canine latissimus dorsi muscle. Circ Res 58:298, 1986.
13. Pette D, Vrbova G: Neural control of phenotypic expression in mammalian muscle fibers. Muscle Nerve 8:676, 1985.
14. Dewar ML, Drinkwater DC, Wittnich C, et al: Synchronously stimulated skeletal muscle graft for myocardial repair. An experimental study. J Thorac Cardiovasc Surg 87:325, 1984.
15. Moreira LFP, Chagas ACP, Camarano GP, et al: Cardiomyoplasty benefits in experimental myocardial dysfunction. J Cardiac Surg 4:164, 1989.
16. Moreira LFP, Chagas ACP, Camarano GP, et al: Bases experimentais da utilização da cardiomioplastia no tratamento da insuficiência miocárdica. Rev Bras Circ Cardiovasc 3:9, 1988.
17. Fragomeni LS, Kaye MP: The registry of the international society for heart transplantation: fifth official report—1988. J Heart Transplantation 7:249, 1988.
18. Baumgartner WA, Augustine S, Borkon AM, et al: Present expectations in cardiac transplantation. Ann Thorac Surg 43:585, 1987.
19. Cançado JR, Chuster M: Cardiopatia Chagásica. Belo Horizonte, I. Oficial, 1985.
20. Chachques JC, Grandjean PA, Carpentier A: Latissimus dorsi dynamic cardiomyoplasty. Ann Thorac Surg 47:600, 1989.
21. Copeland JG, Emery RW, Levinson MM, et al: Selection of patients for cardiac transplantation. Circulation 75:2, 1987.
22. Mannion JD, Velchik MA, Acker MA, et al: Transmural blood flow of multi-layered latissimus dorsi skeletal muscle ventricles during circulatory assistance. Trans Am Soc Artif Intern Organs 32:454, 1986.
23. Ballester M, Jajoo J, Rees S, et al: The mechanism of mitral regurgitation in dilated left ventricle. Clin Cardiol 6:333, 1983.
24. Stevenson LW, Perloff JK: The dilated cardiomyopathies: clinical aspects. Cardiol Clin 6:187, 1988.
25. Moreira LFP, Stolf NAG, Jatene AD: Hemodynamic benefits of cardiomyoplasty in clinical and experimental myocardial dysfunction. In RC-J Chiu, I Bourgeois (ed.): Transformed Muscle for Cardiac Assist and Repair. Mount Kisco, NY, Futura Publishing Co, 1990, pp 179–188.
26. Anderson WA, Andersen JS, Acker MA, et al: Skeletal muscle grafts applied to the heart. A word of caution. Circulation 78(suppl III):III 180, 1988.

Part III
Experimental Models and Future Developments

Chapter 15

Experimental Cardiomyoplasty with Nerve Stimulation

Manfred Frey, Helmut Gruber, W. Happak, Herwig Thoma*

The first clinical application of dynamic cardiomyoplasty was reported by Carpentier and Chachques in 1985.[1] This success was the result of the increased knowledge together with numerous experiments from various groups of chronic electrostimulation of skeletal muscles for the purpose of partial replacement of heart function and the development of appropriate implantable stimulation devices.

In a previous experimental study in sheep we demonstrated that even large limb muscles like the psoas muscle can be completely transformed to a slow and fatigue-resistant muscle by electrostimulation with low frequency and thus may be applicable as an energy source for implantable artificial organs.[2] However, it is still a long way from stimulating a transformed fatigue-resistant muscle to the energy supply of an artificial heart with this kind of muscle energy. The direct application of the stimulated latissimus dorsi muscle avoids several technical problems such as the transformation of the energy of the muscle contraction to electrical or hydraulic energy for driving an artificial heart.

Therefore, we decided to apply our experience with indirect electrostimulation over multiple epineural electrodes to an experimental model of dynamic cardiomyoplasty in sheep.

Material and Methods

The neurovascular pedicled latissimus dorsi (LD) muscle was used for dynamic cardiomyoplasty in adult sheep (Fig. 1). After the left LD muscle had been dissected free from its origins, the heart was accessed by a lateral tho-

*With the cooperation of G Burggasser, W Mayr, U Losert, M Deutinger, and M Windberger

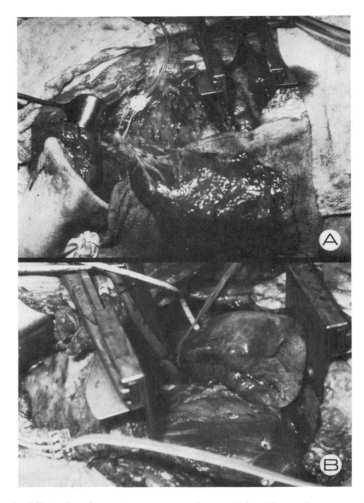

Figure 1. *A. LD isolated on its neurovascular pedicle. Electrodes are sutured to the nerve. B. cardiomyoplasty completed.*

racotomy and a window was created by resection of the lateral part of the second rib. The LD was introduced through this window into the thorax and was wrapped around the whole circumference of both ventricles of the heart. The LD muscle was sutured to the myocardium without cardiopulmonary bypass. As a result, the whole circumference of the heart was covered by skeletal muscle, which was sutured to itself again to provide a complete contracting functional envelope for both ventricles. Four electrodes for stimulation were fixed at the epineurium of the thoracodorsal nerve rather proximally outside the thorax where the mechanical stress for the electrodes was minimal.

Three different groups were studied:

1. Eight acute experiments for standardization of the experimental model.

At first we tried to reduce the heart function by resection of the superficial part of the anterior wall of the left ventricle before cardiomyoplasty. However, we had to return to cardiomyoplasty to the healthy heart as described above mainly because of insurmountable difficulties with the extracorporal circulation in sheep.

2. In three animals the LD muscle was wrapped around the heart without preconditioning and remained there for 3, 4, and 28 days before the final experiments were performed.

3. In three sheep, the LD muscles had been stimulated chronically for 10 weeks prior to transposition (indirect stimulation by implanted stimulators, stimulus amplitude transcutaneously adjusted for achieving vigorous visible contractions, pulse trains of 500-ms length and 15-Hz frequency with intervals of 1 sec). Muscle biopsies at 2 weeks showed the degree of transformation of fast muscle fibers to slow fatigue-resistant fibers for preconditioning. Cardiomyoplasty was performed after 10 weeks, because transformation was comlete at that time. The final experiments became necessary 63 and 144 days after transposition of the preconditioned latissimus dorsi muscle.

In groups 2 and 3 stimulation was continued 1 week after transposition and adjusted to contraction levels that did not impede cardiac circulatory function.

In the final experiments, the influence of the transposed LD muscle on functional parameters of the heart was tested with stimulation on and off. The effect was evaluated for stimulation triggered optimally by the ECG or applied asynchronously to the heart action.

All muscle biopsies taken during and at the end of the experiments were frozen in 2-methylbutane at $-80°C$ and transverse cryostat sections were stained for hematoxylin-eosin (HE), actomyosin ATPase after alkaline (pH 10.4) and acid preincubation (pH 4.3),[3] and NDH-TR.[4] Sections stained for ATPase (pH 4.3) were evaluated by computer-assisted image analysis in respect to muscle fiber diameters of type I and type II fibers. Statistical parameters and distribution histograms were printed out. HE-stained sections were qualitatively analyzed in regard to endomyseal edema, fat tissue, and degenerating and regenerating muscle fibers. For demonstration of the connective tissue at the contact surface between LD and epicardium, formaldehyde-fixed tissue blocks were embedded in Paraplast and sections were stained for van Gieson.

Results

The results are summarized in the following paragraphs.

· Transposition of the LD results in a heavy ischemic and operative trauma to the muscle (Fig. 2A,B).
· Recovery from this trauma to the muscle during transposition requires 3–4 weeks (Fig. 2C)—the time necessary for the numerous necrotic muscle fibers to regenerate.
· Epineural electrostimulation for 10 weeks makes a complete transformation of type II fibers to slow type I fibers (Fig. 3).

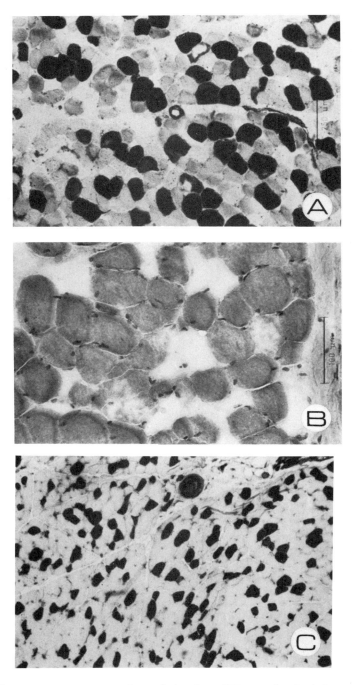

Figure 2. *Transverse cryostat sections of the sheep LD muscle: A. 4 days after transposition to the heart showing endomysial edema and necrosis of muscle fibers, ATPase staining, and acid preincubation. B. Higher magnification of A, HE staining. C. 4 weeks after transposition, recovery from ischemic trauma, muscle fibers regenerated, ATPase, and acid preincubation.*

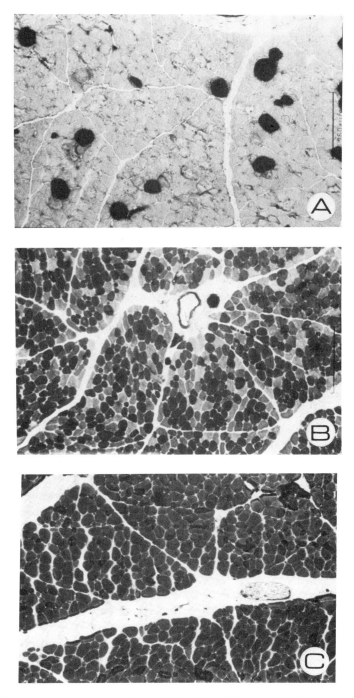

Figure 3. *Transverse cryostat sections of the sheep LD muscle, ATPase staining, and acid preincubation: A. Normal LD. B. Partial transformation to type I fibers after preconditioning stimulation for 4 weeks. C. Complete transformation after stimulation for 10 weeks.*

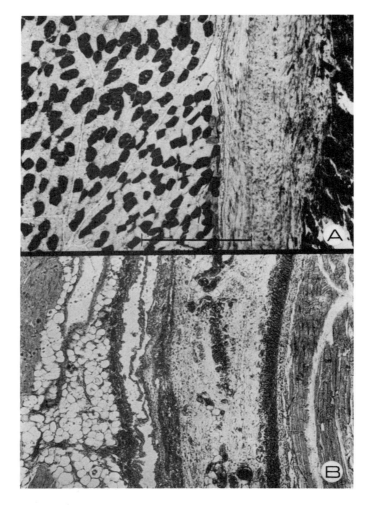

Figure 4. *Transverse cryostat sections at the border between LD and heart: thin layer of loose, gliding connective tissues. A. ATPase staining and acid preincubation. B. van Gieson staining.*

· The effect of preconditioning is partly lost during the postoperative period without stimulation.
· Only a thin layer of loose connective tissue is built up between skeletal muscle and epicardium (Fig. 4).
· There is pronounced scarring between the LD muscle and the thoracic wall. Contraction of the stimulated latissimus dorsi muscle can be limited by this scarring.
· The missing experimental model for reduction of the heart function makes estimation of functional efficiency of cardiomyoplasty in animals difficult. The application of cardiomyoplasty to the healthy heart will

not result in a positive functional influence of the stimulated skeletal muscle to the heart.

Asynchronous stimulation of LD muscle or inadequate length of pulse trains causes arrhythmia and extrasystoles.

Discussion

Indirect stimulation of the LD muscle by multiple steel-electrodes fixed to the epineurium of the thoracodorsal nerve outside the thorax reduces mechanical stress on the electrodes during muscle contraction. The electrodes around the thoracodorsal nerve are easily accessed through the fat pad of the axilla.

If the electrodes have to be replaced, the thorax does not have to be reopened. Using microsurgical techniques, the small electrodes are removed easily from the epineurium without harm to the nerve. New electrodes can be sutured to another segment of the nerve for replacement if necessary.

Using indirect stimulation, a more physiological, rotating multichannel stimulation becomes applicable with less fatigue.

A very selective stimulation of the latissimus dorsi muscle becomes possible over multiple electrodes. The best pattern of muscle contraction with the optimal function benefit can be selected by optimal combination of the activated electrodes.

If one of the electrodes malfunctions, it can be removed from the rotating activation since the other working electrodes guarantee the continuation of functional stimulation.

After transposition to the heart the LD muscle requires approximately 3 weeks for good recovery from the ischemic trauma. Stimulation should not be started too early.

The preconditioning effect is partially lost during the recovery phase without stimulation. Preconditioning seems not to be of real importance for clinical application due to the long period needed for the regeneration of necrotic muscle fibers before electrostimulation can be started again.

Scarring, which limits the excursion of muscle contraction, is minimal between the LD and the heart (danger of luxation of the heart out of the muscle pouch) and much more between the LD and the thoracic wall. This can be prevented by interposition of the pericardium.

It is not possible to derive any conclusions on the functional improvement in this experimental model because the LD muscle is wrapped around a normally functioning heart. However, this study does show that stimulation of the nerve instead of the muscle is an efficient alternative in cardiomyoplasty.

References

1. Carpentier A, Chachques JC: Successful cardiomyoplasty with an electrostimulated latissimus dorsi flap. Proceedings 14th Meeting of the Euroelectric Society, Int. Symposium on Biomechanics of Muscle, Athens, p. 27, 1985.

2. Frey M, Thoma H, Gruber H, et al: The chronically stimulated muscle as an energy source for artificial organs. Eur Surg Res 16:232, 1984.
3. Guth L, Samaha FJ: Procedure for the histochemical demonstration of actomyosin ATPase. Exp Eurol 28:365, 1970.
4. Dubowitz V: Muscle Biopsy: A Practice Approach. London, Philadelphia, Toronto, Baelliere Tindall, 1985.

Chapter 16

Cardiomyoplasty at a High Heart Rate

Yoshihiro Naruse, Tatsuhiko Takahama, Akira Furuse

Tachycardia is one of the most serious problems of dynamic cardiomyoplasty. Contraction of the heart can be disturbed by the skeletal muscle sutured to the heart when both ventricles are wrapped by the skeletal muscle. This chapter is a discussion of our investigation of the efficacy of dynamic cardiomyoplasty at a heart rate >100 bpm in six dogs.

Methods

In six anesthetized open-chest dogs, both ventricles were wrapped by the dissected left latissimus dorsi (LD) muscle that had been electrically preconditioned for more than 6 weeks (Fig. 1).

While monitoring pressures of the descending aorta (AOP) and the main pulmonary artery (PAP), LD muscle was stimulated synchronously (synchronization rate 1:1 and 3:1) with variable heart rates of more than 100 bpm.

The left ventricular volume was measured in each animal with a volume conductance catheter developed by Baan et al. and the left ventricular pressure was measured with a catheter-tip transducer (Millar).

End-systolic pressure volume relationship (ESPVR) was determined from multiple pressure volume loops obtained during brief preload reduction by balloon occlusion of the inferior vena cava.

Results

In all animals, synchronous contraction of the LD muscle produced an increase in the systolic left ventricular pressure and a decrease in the left

From *Cardiomyoplasty* edited by Alain Carpentier, MD, PhD, Juan-Carlos Chachques, MD, and Pierre Grandjean, MS © 1991. Futura Publishing Inc., Mount Kisco, NY.

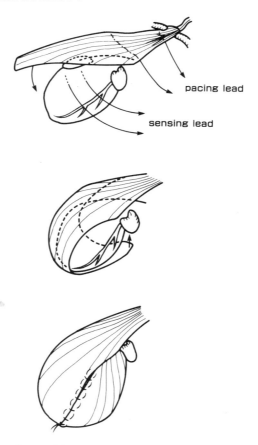

Figure 1. *The preconditioned latissimus dorsi was dissected and sutured around both ventricles. Two pacing leads were attached to the muscle, and two sensing electrodes were fixed to the right ventricle.*

ventricular end-systolic volume without elevation of the left ventricular end-diastolic pressure up to a heart rate of 120 bpm.

When the LD muscle was stimulated, the pressure volume loops shifted to the left and the slope of ESPVR increased significantly (Fig. 2).

At a heart rate of 130 bpm, a distinct systolic augmentation of the AOP was not always seen with 1.1 synchronization. When the synchronization rate was 3:1, systolic AOP was improved by stimulation even at the same heart rate.

Systolic augmentation of PAP occurred up to a rate of 150 bpm even with 1:1 synchronization. Above 130 bpm, the systolic PAP appeared to increase more significantly with3:1 synchronization than with 1:1 synchronization.

Figure 3 represents systolic augmentation of AOP and PAP produced by 3:1 synchronous stimulation. Systolic pressures of both AOP and PAP increased significantly when the LD muscle was stimulated.

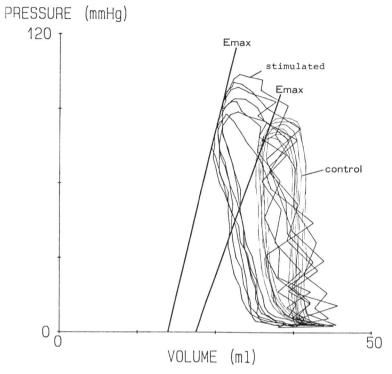

Figure 2. *Pressure-volume data from a dog after cardiomyoplasty (heart rate 120 bpm, 1:1 synchronization). Muscle stimulation produced an increase in the slope of end-systolic pressure-volume relationship.*

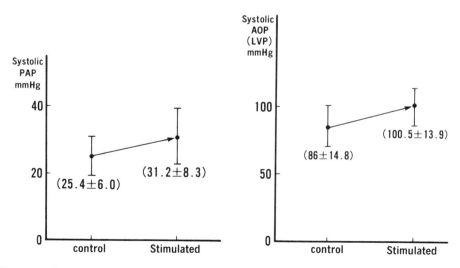

Figure 3. *Systolic augmentation produced by contraction of the latissimus dorsi muscle with 3:1 synchronization. AOP = aortic pressure; PAP = pulmonary artery pressure.*

Comment

Although the efficacy of dynamic cardiomyoplasty has not been clearly determined, increase in the slope of ESPVR evidently shows that left ventricular contractility was improved by synchronous contraction of the LD muscle. At a heart rate above 120 bpm, cardiac contraction may be affected by the stimulated skeletal muscle with 1:1 synchronization. Under this condition, stimulation with 3:1 synchronization was considered to be effective for cardiac assist.

Chapter 17

Atriomyoplasty in the Fontan Procedure

Didier Loulmet, Alain Carpentier, Regent L. Beaudet

Cavopulmonary derivation is based on the principle that the right ventricle is not essential for adequate pulmonary perfusion.[1] It consists of directing blood flow from the right atrium to the pulmonary artery, thus bypassing the right ventricle. The negligible contraction of the right atrium and the absence of valves between the vena cava and the right atrium causes the pulmonary flow to be continuous rather than pulsatile. Flow through the lungs is assured by a pressure gradient between the right and the left atria.[2] In 1986, Carpentier et al. extended the concept of cardiomyoplasty to the Fontan operation in a patient who had an atriopulmonary correction and who 6 years later developed high pulmonary resistance (unpublished data). The aim was to reinforce right atrial contraction to restore pulsatile flow in the pulmonary artery and to increase the pressure gradient between the two atria. This concept had been investigated in preliminary experiments using the right latissimus dorsi (RLD) muscle, but results showed little change in the hemodynamic parameters.[3] In order to improve the result, Carpentier suggested the use of the left latissimus dorsi and separation of the two atria by extensive dissection of the interatrial groove. The extremity of the latissimus dorsi is secured to the bottom of this interatrial trench so as to circumscribe most of the right atrium (Fig. 1). This paper reports the experimental results obtained with this new technique.

Material and Methods

Three dogs were anesthetized with IV sodium pentobartibal (30 mg/kg). Mechanical ventilation was used throughout the experiment except during cardiopulmonary bypass (CPB). Animals were monitored by hematocrit and serial blood gas determinations. The left femoral artery was cannulated for

From *Cardiomyoplasty* edited by Alain Carpentier, MD, PhD, Juan-Carlos Chachques, MD, and Pierre Grandjean, MS © 1991. Futura Publishing Inc., Mount Kisco, NY.

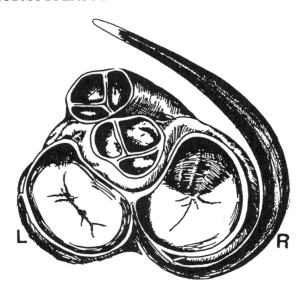

Figure 1. *Carpentier technique using the left latissimus dorsi muscle and extensive separation of the interatrial groove.*

monitoring of the arterial pressure. Following median sternotomy, the azygos vein was ligated and both vena cava were encircled. Heparin was administered (100 IU/kg). CPB was set between the vena cava and the right femoral artery. The inferior vena cava was cannulated via the right femoral vein so as to facilitate the valve implantation at the junction of the right atrium and the inferior vena cava. Atriopulmonary derivation was performed before starting CPB: a vascular graft (18 m Vascutek vascular graft, Medtronic) was anastomosed between the right atrial appendage and the main pulmonary artery. The graft was left clamped until later in the experiment, and CPB then was started. The caval tapes were tied and the inferior vena cava was clamped as close as possible to the diaphragm. Following right atrial opening, the tricuspid orifice was closed by suturing the annulus thus excluding the right ventricle. A mechanical valve (Medtronic-Hall) was inserted into each vena cava. The right atrium was closed by a running suture and the atriopulmonary shunt unclamped. CPB was terminated in the usual manner. Sodium bicarbonate was administered to adjust pH, and filling pressure was modulated with a lactate Ringer's solution. During the period of hemodynamic stabilization, the left latissimus dorsi (LLD) muscle was mobilized and brought into the chest through a left thoracotomy at the level of the fifth intercostal space. The interatrial groove was dissected and the distal part of the LLD muscle was sutured within the dissected interatrial groove so as to cover most of the right atrium. Electrodes of stimulation were placed directly on the thoracodorsal nerve and the stimulation was performed with a variable parameter burst generator (S48 stimulator, Grass Instrument). The muscle was not preconditioned, and the stimulation was not synchronized with the heart contraction.

The stimulation protocol used a burst frequency of 30 Hz and an ON-OFF cycle of 250 ms–750 ms. Stimulation was begun immediately after muscle implantation. Catheters were inserted into the pulmonary artery and the inferior vena cava. Hemodynamic data was recorded on a multichannel recorder (7758 A recorder, Hewlett-Packard).

Results

After atriopulmonary derivation, satisfactory hemodynamics could be maintained. All dogs were in sinus rhythm. No atrioventricular conduction block occurred. Moderate distension of the right atrium was observed. Without stimulation, pressure tracings showed that the flow pattern in the pulmonary artery had lost its normal pulsatile waveform. Hemodynamic changes observed at the time of stimulation are shown in Figure 2. The LLD muscle contraction generated a pulmonary wave of pressure in each dog reaching an average pic of 33 ± 5.8 mm Hg. No decrease in inferior vena cava pressure was observed probably because of the short duration of the experiments.

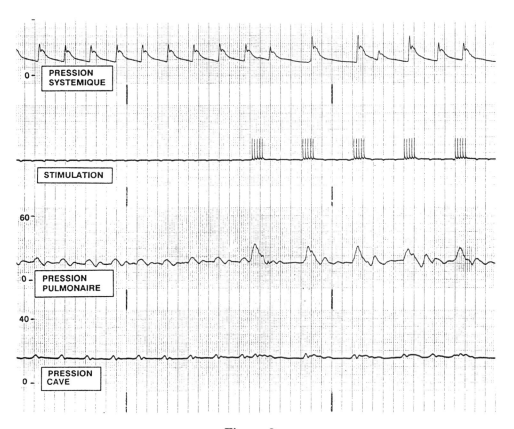

Figure 2.

Discussion

Tricuspid atresia was simulated in dogs by closing the tricuspid orifice. The pulmonary valve was not closed in order to avoid a right ventricular distension by direct intraventricular venous return. Pulmonary flow was maintained by a vascular graft inserted between the right atrium and the pulmonary artery. This model enabled us to obtain a good proxy for a functional exclusion of the right ventricle.[4] Hemodynamic measurements showed a pattern of continuous pressure identical to the pattern obtained after a Fontan operation with negligible effect from the right atrial contraction. To maximize the effect of the right atrial contraction we used the contraction of the LLD muscle induced by a myostimulator. Valves were inserted into the two vena cavae to assure a unidirectional flow. A valve was not placed in the atriopulmonary tube, which may have further improved the efficiency of the operation. Pressure recordings indicated that muscle stimulation restored a pulsatile pattern of pressure in the pulmonary artery. Results obtained with LLD muscle were superior to those obtained in our previous experiments using the RLD muscle because the former permits a larger coverage of the right atrium and a better orientation of the muscle. Although encouraging, these results are not conclusive because the pulmonary flow could not be recorded and no decrease in the pressure of the inferior vena cava was observed. These two elements will be further investigated in future experiments.

References

1. Sade R, Castaneda A: The dispensable right ventricle. Surgery 77:624, 1975.
2. Main D, Rice M, Hagler D, et al: Outcome of the Fontan procedure in patients with tricuspid atresia. Circulation Suppl II:88, 1985.
3. Loulmet D, Comtois A, Hollmann C, et al: Application of cardiomyoplasty to the Fontan operation: hemodynamic observations. In RC-J Chiu, IM Bourgeois (eds). Transformed Muscle for Cardiac Assist and Repair. Mount Kisco, NY, Futura Publishing Co, 1990, pp 247–251.
4. Chachques JC, Grandjean PA, Pfeffer TA, et al: Cardiac assistance by atrial or ventricular cardiomyoplasty. J Heart Transplant 9:239, 1990.

Chapter 18

Dynamic Aortomyoplasty

Juan-Carlos Chachques, Pierre A. Grandjean, Alain Carpentier

We investigated the use of the patient's own skeletal muscles to augment myocardial performance. Dynamic cardiomyoplasty has demonstrated experimentally and clinically its capacity to chronically improve ventricular function.[1-4] Other works conducted approximately during the same time period have investigated the use of hydraulic pouches powered by rectus, latissimus dorsi, or diaphragm muscles stimulated following a counterpulsation mode.[5-7] The aim of dynamic aortomyoplasty is to create a new hemocompatible contractile chamber from the ascending aorta after enlarging its diameter with an autologous pericardial patch. The ascending aorta is then wrapped with a latissimus dorsi muscle flap (LDMF) electrostimulated in a counterpulsation manner. The left ventricular afterload is thus more effectively decreased, and the counterpulsation is carried out at the vicinity of the coronary artery ostia.

The advantages of dynamic aortomyoplasty using the ascending aorta rather than the descending aorta are: (1) it avoids paraplegia due to spinal cord ischemia; (2) it benefits from the larger diameter of the ascending aorta, which provides a larger volume of blood.

Another modality is to place a biological valve distal to the aortomyoplasty and just before the site of implantation of the brachiocephalic trunk. This biomechanical device acts like a new ventricle with the impaired left ventricle serving as a second atrium.

Material and Methods

Eight adult alpine goats weighing 36 to 45 kg were used. Anesthesia was induced with an intramuscular injection of xylazine 2% and maintained with IV alfaxalonum-alfadolon. All goats underwent a right vertical lateral thoracic incision to facilitate the dissection of the latissimus dorsi (LD) muscle. The right LD muscle was divided from its insertion on the lateral aspect of the last four ribs, iliac crest, and thoracolumbar fascia and mobilized proximally as a

From *Cardiomyoplasty* edited by Alain Carpentier, MD, PhD, Juan-Carlos Chachques, MD, and Pierre Grandjean, MS © 1991. Futura Publishing Inc., Mount Kisco, NY.

pedicle flap. Two pacing electrodes (Medtronic Model SP5528) were implanted into the proximal part of the muscle flap, which was brought into the chest through an opening made by resecting a portion of the second rib. Care was taken to preserve the neurovascular bundle (Fig. 1).

Sternotomy was performed. The ascending aorta and the transverse aortic arch and its branches were dissected (Fig. 1A). In four goats, the ascending aorta was enlarged by implantation of an elliptical patch of autologous pericardium treated with glutaraldehyde. This was done by side clamping of the aorta and polypropylene monofilament 5–0 continuous suture (Fig. 1B). The intraoperative treatment of the pericardium patch with a glutaraldehyde solution (0.62%, 10 min minimum immersion time) allows sufficient collagen cross-linking to ensure pericardial stability in high-pressure circulatory areas.[8]

The ascending and transverse aorta was then wrapped with the latissimus dorsi muscle flap (LDMF) in a counterclockwise fashion, so that its fibers were perpendicular to the longitudinal axis of the aorta. In order to cover the aorta at both sides of the brachiocephalic trunk, the distal end of the LDMF was split longitudinally (Figs. 1C-D), taking into account its intramuscular neurovascular anatomy.[9] The proximity of the ascending aorta with the right LDMF allowed the positioning of the better contractile segment of the muscle (middle segment) in direct contact with the enlarged aorta.

Skeletal muscle electrostimulation was performed using an external counterpulsator (Medtronic Model SP3076) connected to a sensing myocardial lead (Medtronic Model SP5548) and to LDMF pacing electrodes. Muscle stimulation parameters were the following: pulse amplitude 4–6 V, pulse width 0.2 ms, burst rate 30 Hz, and burst duration 185 ms. Diastolic counterpulsation was performed using a delay from the R wave adjusted to provide optimal diastolic augmentation. Short-term cyclic skeletal muscle electrostimulation (10 min/cycle) was delivered to functionally study dynamic aortomyoplasty.

Hemodynamic parameters studies included LV, aortic, and pulmonary pressures and dP/dt. The extent of diastolic augmentation was measured by the subendocardial viability index: diastolic pressure time index (DPTI) /systolic tension-time index (TTI).[10,11]

Percentage increase in this ratio (DPTI/TTI) was calculated during unassisted and assisted cardiac cycles (1:2) in the basal state and after acute heart failure induced by a high dose of propanolol (3 mg/kg/IV). The subendocardial viability index (DPTI/TTI) was derived from superimposed tracings of aortic arch and LV pressures.

Statistical analysis was performed using paired t-test and analysis of variance. Values reported were mean ± standard deviation. A p value of less than 0.05 was considered statistically significant.

Results

Experimental results were obtained in the acute phase. As expected, muscle fatigability occurs 4 to 6 minutes after induction of stimulation.

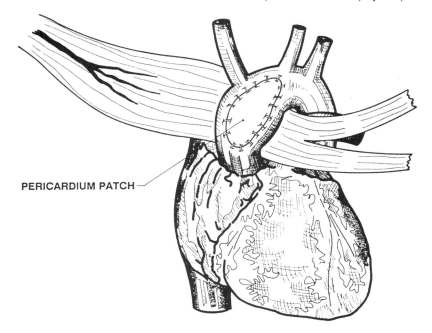

PERICARDIUM PATCH

Figure 1A. *The ascending aorta, the transverse aortic arch and its branches are dissected. The aorta is enlarged by implantation of a patch of autologous pericardium.*

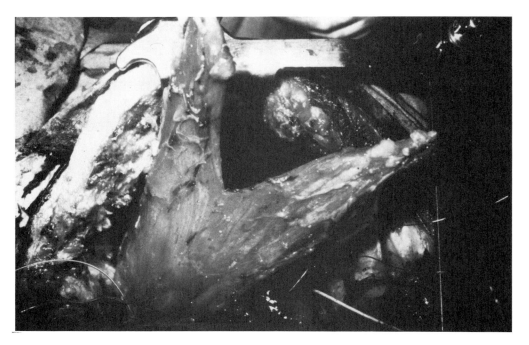

Figure 1B. *The LDMF is positioned behind the aorta, its distal end is split longitudinally.*

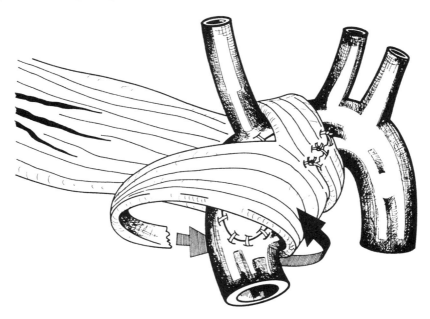

Figure 1C. *The aorta is wrapped by the LDMF in a counterclockwise fashion.*

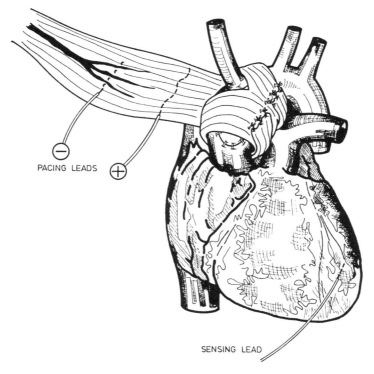

PACING LEADS

SENSING LEAD

Figure 1D. *The aorta is covered at both sides of the brachiocephalic trunk. Muscular fibers lie perpendicular to the longitudinal axis of the aorta.*

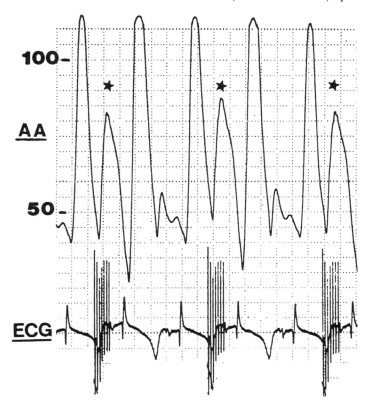

Figure 2. *Hemodynamic recording after dynamic aortomyoplasty. Ascending aorta (AA) pressure in basal conditions. The asterisk (*) marks diastolic augmentation in assisted cycles; heart-to-muscle contraction ratio 2:1.*

The diameter of the ascending aorta in goats was 14.5 ± 3 mm. The surface area of the pericardial aortic patch used in four goats was 260 ± 30 mm². The length of the aortic segment wrapped by the LDMF was 70 ± 8 mm.

The average ascending-aortic peak pressure generated by dynamic aortomyoplasty in basal conditions was 90 mm Hg (systemic blood pressure 115/65mm Hg) (Fig. 2). In the four goats with aortic enlargement, the average peak pressure during LDMF stimulation was 105 mm Hg (systemic pressure: 105/70 mm Hg) (Fig. 3).

Tables 1 and 2 show the hemodynamic data obtained: diastolic aortic counterpulsation by stimulated LDMF resulted in a significant increase of DPTI/TTI both in the basal state conditions (+29.3%) (Fig. 4) and after induced cardiac failure (+26.8%). In the group with aortic enlargement, however, the average increase of DPTI/TTI was +35.8% and +42.2%, respectively.

During these experiments, we noted that the electrostimulated LDMF contracted vigorously. Its mechanical action over the aorta resulted in a homogeneous "systolic activity." No displacement or angularities of the aortic arch and no aortic valve regurgitation were observed. Despite the fact that

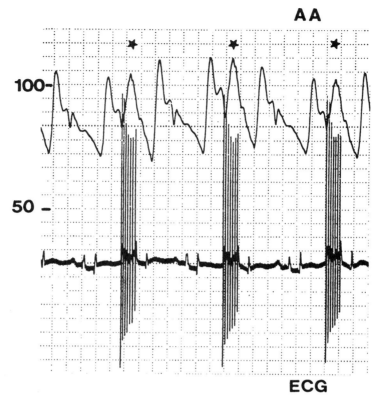

Figure 3. *Diastolic augmentation (*) after ascending aortic (AA) enlargement.*

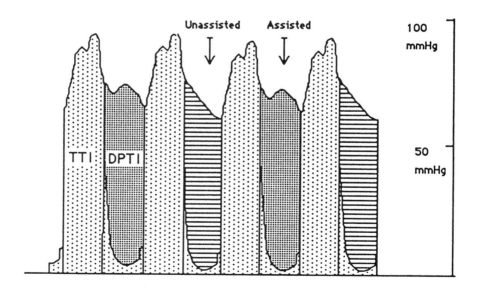

Subendocardial Viability Index : DPTI/TTI

Figure 4. *Increase of subendocardial viability ratio (DPTI/TTI) during assisted cycles after dynamic aortomyoplasty (experiment no. 8, Table 1).*

Table 1
Increase in Subendocardial Viability Index (DPTI/TTI) with Dynamic
Aortomoplasty Diastolic Augmentation on Alternate (2:1) Cardiac Cycles

Experiment	Contol		Cardiac Failure	
	Without St	With St	Without St	With St
1	0.95	1.35	0.98	1.40
3	0.88	1.22	0.86	1.25
6	1.18	1.29	1.08	1.38
7	0.82	1.34	0.84	1.32
2	1.02	1.40	1.05	1.31
4	1.05	1.38	0.99	1.33
5	0.98	1.18	0.95	1.20
8	1.11	1.42	1.00	1.22
$\overline{X}$	0.998	1.322	0.968	1.301
SD	0.117	0.086	0.084	0.072

Paired t-test
(2p)   DF:7   T: -7.339 $p < 0.001$ DF:7   T: -10.283 $p < 0.001$

Table 2
Increase in Subendocardial Viability Index in the Group of Experiments
with Aortic Enlargement

Experiment	Control		Cardiac Failure	
	Without St	With St	Without St	With St
1	0.95	1.35	0.98	1.40
3	0.88	1.22	0.86	1.25
6	1.18	1.29	1.08	1.38
7	0.82	1.34	0.84	1.32
$\overline{X}$	0.957	1.300	0.940	1.337
SD	0.157	0.059	0.112	0.067

Paired t-test
(2p)   DF:3   T: -3.980 $P < 0.05$ DF:3   T: -10.6 $p < 0.005$

heparin was not used during these experiments, no thrombus was noted in the aortic chambers.

Discussion

Although dynamic cardiomyoplasty has already shown promising results in the human,[3] our interest in dynamic aortomyoplasty was stimulated by its possible use as a complementary technique. In this technique, the native ascending aorta, enlarged by an autologous pericardial patch, contracts in a counterpulsation mode. Since no foreign nor synthetic materials are used, this technique avoids thrombotic complications and systemic emboli observed in skeletal muscle-powered neo-ventricles using prosthetic chambers.[11-14]

Skeletal muscle plasticity and its adaptative changes is the basic physiological concept of biomechanical assist devices. The efficacy of skeletal muscle contractile force to augment left ventricular function has been documented experimentally and clinically by the cardiomyoplasty procedure.[1-3,15] Electrical induction of fatigue resistance in skeletal muscles may also be adequately effective for chronic circulatory assistance using diastolic counterpulsation. The aortomyoplasty represents a search for a biomechanical extracardiac circulatory assist device in conjunction with a cardiomyoplasty or in cases where cardiomyoplasty is not possible (extremely dilated cardiomyopathies) or contraindicated (previous cardiac operations, mitral valve insufficiency, hypertrophic cardiomyopathies).

Results obtained with induced cardiac failure showed that when the aorta is enlarged the increase in subendocardial viability index is larger than when the aorta is left intact. It means that a dilated ventricle is better assisted by larger aortic chamber volume.

Patients with a large ascending aorta will probably not require such a patch enlargement of the aorta. Aortic valve regurgitation, Marfan's syndrome, as well as calcified ascending aorta are contraindications for dynamic aortomyoplasty. Routine preoperative CT scan and NMR would be indicated to detect aortic calcifications in candidates prior to surgery. On a hypothetical basis, dynamic aortomyoplasty can be viewed as a complementary technique in patients who have undergone left ventricular cardiomyoplasty and in whom a supplementary hemodynamic support is required.

The extensive experience with intra-aortic balloon pump (IABP) demonstrated considerable hemodynamic and physiological benefits of diastolic counterpulsation to the failing heart.[16] Extra-aortic ventricles wrapped with electrostimulated muscles[17] were as effective in this regard but led to thromboembolic complications resulting from blood-artificial surface interactions. Dynamic aortomyoplasty might be viewed as a potential permanent perivascular assist device.

Although short-term experimental dynamic aortomyoplasty led to a significant diastolic augmentation, a long-term study using this procedure will allow us to evaluate the hemodynamic and functional effect of this biomechanical assist device to support chronic ventricular failure. The muscle looses some of its blood supply, and hence, we assume that postoperatively its efficiency would be reduced. However, after a delay (2 weeks), sufficient blood flow is re-established by means of collateral circulation and muscle function will recover. On the other hand, it is also important to consider postoperative muscle training. Chronically electrostimulated skeletal muscle undergoes metabolic transformation (glycolytic toward oxidative) with induction of fatigue resistance.[18,19]

Before it can be used in the clinical setting, upcoming experimental studies of dynamic aortomyoplasty should answer the following questions:

1. What are the effects of long-term diastolic counterpulsation?
2. What is the potential deleterious effect of an aortomyoplasty on the aorta?
3. What are the long-term advantages of aortomyoplasty over muscle-powered pouches?

We think these questions are partially clarified by the circulatory regimen of the kangaroo[20] in which the ascending aorta pressure waveform displays a very large secondary wave that begins in late systole or early diastole and continues throughout most of diastole. The peak of this secondary wave (which almost always occurs in diastole) is often greater than systolic peak pressure and apparently results from intense wave reflections from peripheral vascular beds of the lower part of the kangaroo's body. These findings are explicable on the basis of body size and shape and the extreme eccentric location of the heart within the body. This permanent physiological counterpulsationlike system is very well tolerated and assists chronically the voluminous lower part of the kangaroo's body.

Long-term experimental studies involving dynamic aortomyoplasty will elucidate the future and clinical feasibility of this new promising approach to biomechanical assisted circulation.

References

1. Chachques JC, Mitz V, Hero M, et al: Experimental cardiomyoplasty using the latissimus dorsi muscle flap.J Cardiovasc Surg 26:457, 1985.
2. Carpentier A, Chachques JC: Myocardial substitution with a stimulated skeletal muscle: first successful clinical case. Lancet i:1267, 1985.
3. Carpentier A, Chachques JC: The use of stimulated skeletal muscle to replace diseased human heart muscle. Clinical experience. In RC-J Chiu, I Bourgeois (eds): Biomechanical Cardiac Assist: Cardiomyoplasty and Muscle-Powered Devices. Mount Kisco, NY, Futura Publishing Co, 1986, pp 85–102.
4. Chachques JC, Grandjean PA, Schwartz K, et al: Effect of latissimus dorsi dynamic cardiomyoplasty on ventricular function.Circulation 78(suppl 3):203, 1988.
5. Kantrowitz A, McKinnon WMP: The experimental use of the diaphragm as an auxiliary myocardium. Surg Forum 9:266, 1959.
6. Mannion JD, Hammond R, Stephenson LW: Hydraulic pouches of canine latissimus dorsi. J Thorac Cardiovasc Surg 91:534, 1986.
7. Chachques JC, Grandjean PA, Bourgeois I, et al: Dynamic cardiomyoplasty to im-

prove ventricular function. In F Unger (ed): Assisted Circulation. Heidelberg, Springer Verlag, 1989, pp 525–541.

8. Chachques JC, Vasseur B, Perier P, et al: A rapid method to stabilize biological materials for cardiovascular surgery. Ann NY Acad Sci 529:184, 1988.

9. Tobin GR, Schusterman M, Peterson GH, et al: The intramuscular neurovascular anatomy of the Latissimus Dorsi muscle: the basis for splitting the flap. Plast Reconstr Surg 67:637, 1981.

10. Buckberg GD, Fixler DE, Archie JP, et al: Experimental subendocardial ischemia in dogs with normal coronary arteries. Circ Res 30:67, 1962.

11. Neilson IR, Brister SJ, Khalafalla AS, et al: Left ventricular assistance in dogs using a skeletal muscle powered device for diastolic augmentation. Heart Transplantation 4: 343, 1985.

12. Kochamba G, Desrosiers C, Dewar M, et al: The muscle-powered dual-chamber counterpulsation: rheologically superior implantable cardiac assist device. Ann Thorac Surg 45:620, 1988.

13. Mannion JD, Acker MA, Hammond RL, et al: Power output of skeletal muscle ventricles in circulation: short-term studies. Circulation 76:155, 1987.

14. Chiu RC-J, Walsh GL, Dewar ML, et al: Implantable extra-aortic balloon assist powered by transformed fatigue-resistant skeletal muscle. J Thorac Cardiovasc Surg 94:694, 1987.

15. Chachques JC, Grandjean PA, Carpentier A: Latissimus dorsi dynamic cardiomyoplasty. Ann Thorac Surg 47:600, 1989.

16. Kantrowitz A: Experimental augmentation of coronary flow by retardation of the arterial pressure pulse. Surgery 34:678, 1953.

17. Acker MA, Anderson WA, Hammond RL, et al: Skeletal muscle ventricles in circulation. J Thorac Cardiovasc Surg 94:163, 1987.

18. Salmons S, Henriksson J: The adaptative response of skeletal muscle to increased use. Muscle Nerve 4:94, 1981.

19. Pette D, Vrbová G: Neural control of phenotypic espression in mammalian muscle fibers. Muscle Nerve 8:676, 1985.

20. Nichols WW, Avolio AP, O'Rourke MF: Ascending aortic impedance patterns in the kangaroo: their explanation and relation to pressure waveforms. Circ Res 59:247, 1986.

Chapter 19

Effect of Pharmacological Agents on the Trained Latissimus Dorsi Muscles†

Maria J.W. Smets, Caroline M.H.B. Lucas, F.H. Van der Veen*

Anesthesia during routine surgical procedures as well as during cardiac surgery usually requires drug administration to relax the muscles for surgical access, to facilitate control of respiration, and to limit the amount of general anesthetics when relaxation itself is not the primary purpose.[1]

The recent development of a new surgical technique, cardiomyoplasty, requires special anesthetic care.[2,3] Obviously, muscle relaxant drugs like cur-alest and pancuronium are contraindicated during surgery in patients depending hemodynamically on cardiac support by dynamic cardiomyoplasty. In these patients, it is essential to identify anesthetics that might affect skeletal muscle contractility to avoid a decrease in cardiac output. The effect of drugs frequently used during surgery like halothane, lidocaine, fentanyl, midazolam, and propranolol on skeletal muscle contractility is not known because of the lack of an adequate model for testing these drugs.[4,5]

We recently reported an in vivo model in dogs to study latissimus dorsi muscle contractility.[6] This model was used to study the effect of the drugs mentioned above. The experiments were performed in dogs following 12 weeks of latissimus dorsi muscle stimulation to determine the effect of these drugs on trained skeletal muscle. This mimics the clinical situation when cardiomyoplasty patients are undergoing anesthesia because of surgery.

Methods

Stimulation electrodes (Medtronic SP5528) were implanted in the left latissimus dorsi muscle and connected to an Itrel™ pacemaker in four dogs as

* With the cooperation of O.C.K Penn and HJJ Wellens.
† This work, financially supported by the Netherlands Heart Foundation, was done in collaboration with the Bakken Research Center, Maastricht, The Netherlands.
From *Cardiomyoplasty* edited by Alain Carpentier, MD, PhD, Juan-Carlos Chachques, MD, and Pierre Grandjean, MS © 1991. Futura Publishing Inc., Mount Kisco, NY.

described by Van der Veen et al.[6] The latissimus dorsi muscle was stimulated during a 12-week period to obtain a predominantly type I muscle fiber as demonstrated by muscle biopsies.[7] In short, the LD muscle was stimulated using 30-Hz pulses in bursts of 0.25-sec duration, resulting initially in 30 contractions/min and after 10 weeks in 80 contractions/min.

Experimental Protocol

After the dogs were stimulated for at least 12 weeks, drugs were tested at weekly intervals to avoid possible interaction. On the day of study, dogs were premedicated with a drug mixture (0.2 mL/kg IM) containing per milliliter 10 mg oxycodon HCl, 1 mg acepromazine, 0.5 mg atropine sulphate. Induction followed using 5–7 mg/kg pentobarbital (Narcovet) intravenously.

Subsequently, the dogs were intubated and ventilated with N_2O and O_2. The left front leg was attached to a force displacement transducer (Grass FT 10) according to the method of van der Veen and coworkers.

One of the following drugs was thereafter administered: halothane 0.75%, lidocaine 1 mg/kg IV, and midazolam 0.3 mg/kg IV. These drugs were studied twice in all four dogs and data are presented as n = 8. In addition, fentanyl 5 μg/kg IV, and propranolol 0.2 mg/kg IV as a bolus followed by a 1-hour infusion of 0.1 mg/kg/h were studied separately in the four dogs. These measurements are presented as n = 4.

Muscle contraction was studied during stimulation with bursts (1–sec duration; 8-sec intervals) at a frequency range from 2 to 50 Hz, and the peak force calculated from paper recordings. The duration of each test procedure was approximately 5 minutes, involving at least 3 contractions at 10 different frequencies.

Latissimus dorsi muscle contractility was examined before drug administration and 1 minute after lidocaine; 5, 15, and 25 minutes after fentanyl, halothane, and midazolam; and 5, 30, and 60 minutes following a bolus injection of propranolol. Within these time periods, the plasma concentration of these drugs are assumed to include the peak values.[1,4,5] During the contractility tests of lidocaine and propanolol routine anesthesia was maintained using halothane 0.5 %.

Data are presented as mean and SEM. Changes in force are presented as the percentage of the control value measured just before drug administration on the same day.

Results

Fiber composition of the left latissimus dorsi muscle changed from a 30% to an 80% type I fiber after 12 weeks of electrical stimulation, which is comparable to the findings of Havenith and coworkers.[7]

Lidocaine administration did not affect latissimus dorsi muscle force in the frequency range from 2 to 50 Hz (Fig. 1). There was no effect of fentanyl bolus injection on latissimus dorsi muscle force after 5 minutes. However, a

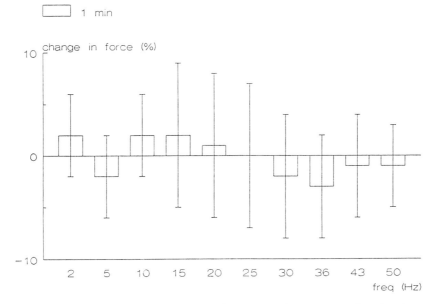

Figure 1. *The relative change of LD muscle contractility measured at 1 minute after administration of lidocaine (1 mg/kg, IV). Measurements were performed at a frequency range from 2 to 50 Hz. n = 8; mean ± SEM*

relatively small negative effect was observed both at 15 and 25 minutes after administration at higher frequencies of 43 and 50 Hz (Fig. 2). Halothane did not change contractile force when measured after 5, 15, and 25 minutes (Fig. 3), although a large variation was observed in comparison to contractile force after fentanyl administration (Fig. 2). Midazolam significantly decreased contractile force at 25 and 30 Hz stimulation after 5, 15, and 25 minutes of administration (Fig. 4). A consistent decrease of about 9% at 30 Hz during at least 25 minutes was observed. Propranolol reduced contractile force during at least 1 hour following its administration (Fig. 5). In particular, at 30 Hz a decrease of 27% was observed after 30 minutes.

Discussion

In situ skeletal muscle stimulation in dogs as used in this study appears to be a sensitive model to examine the effect of drugs on skeletal muscle contractile force. The large variety of drugs routinely used during cardiomyoplasty or general surgery necessitates the evaluation of the effect of these drugs on skeletal muscle contractility.[2,3,8–10]

Force measurements were started 1 minute after lidocaine bolus injection because a cardiac effect can be observed after 1–2 minutes. Although a large variation in contractile force was observed during the test procedure, our ob-

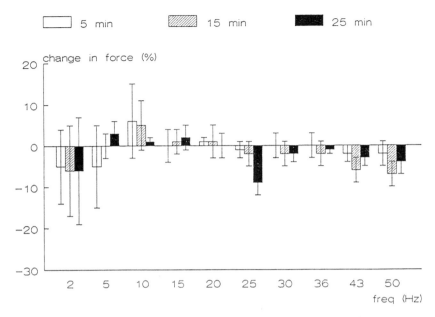

Figure 2. *The relative change of LD muscle contractility measured at 5, 15, and 25 minutes after fentanyl administration (5 µg/kg IV). n = 4*

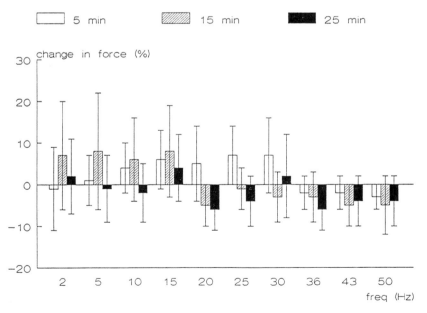

Figure 3. *The relative change of LD muscle contractility measured at 5, 15, and 25 minutes after halothane administration (0.75%). n = 8*

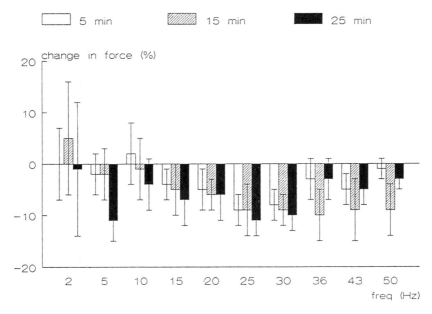

Figure 4. *The relative change of LD muscle contractility measured at 5, 15, and 25 minutes after midazolam administration (0.3 mg/kg). n = 8*

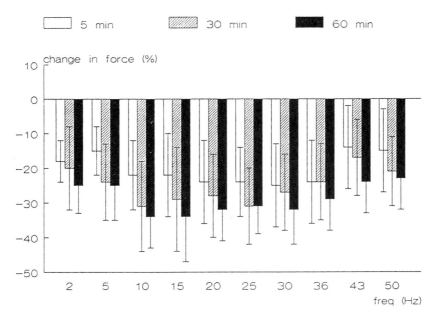

Figure 5. *The relative change of LD muscle contractility measured at 5, 30, and 60 minutes after propranolol administration. The dosage used was an initial bolus of 0.2 mg/kg intravenously following by an infusion of 0.1 mg/kg/h. n = 4*

servations suggest that lidocaine can be used safely after cardiomyoplasty in a therapeutic dosage of 1 mg/kg.

Our study did not show a significant effect of fentanyl on skeletal muscle contractile force at a therapeutic dosage of 5 μg/kg. This implies that fentanyl can be used after cardiomyoplasty if muscle relaxing drugs are omitted. In addition, halothane did not affect skeletal muscle contractility until approximately 25 minutes after its administration.

The use of midazolam after cardiomyoplasty should be limited because skeletal muscle contractility decreased significantly (10%) at 30 Hz at 25 minutes after administration.

Propranolol had a pronounced negative effect on latissimus dorsi muscle contractile force and decreased contractility with approximately 30% at 30 Hz. This suggests that the long-lasting negative effect of propranolol on cardiac muscle contractility runs parallel to skeletal muscle contractility reduction.

A decrease of skeletal muscle contractility after drug administration has major implications during a cardiomyoplasty procedure and during general surgery in patients who had the cardiomyoplasty procedure in the past. First, contractile properties of the LD muscle are investigated using test stimuli when the muscle is dissected free and stimulation electrodes are placed. Results of these measurements are then used to program the Cardiomyostimulator™ Pulse Train Generator during the subsequent period of cardiac assist.[3] Second, drugs that reduce skeletal muscle contractility decrease cardiac pump function in patients who are hemodynamically depending on dynamic cardiomyoplasty as reported by Chachques and coworkers.[2]

Halothane, lidocaine, and fentanyl can be used safely during anesthesia following cardiomyoplasty. Administration of midazolam should be limited because it reduces skeletal muscle contractility force. The use of propranolol should be avoided because a severe decrease of trained latissimus dorsi muscle contractility does occur.

References

1. Churchill-Davidson HC (ed): Wylie and Churchill-Davidson's A Practise of Anesthesia. London, Lloyd-Luke, 1978.
2. Chachques JC, Grandjean P, Schwartz K, et al: Effect of latissimus dorsi dynamic cardiomyoplasty on ventricular function. Circulation 78:III203, 1988.
3. Molteni L, Almada H, Ferreira R: Synchronously stimulated skeletal muscle graft for left ventricular assistance. J Thorac Cardiovasc Surg 97:439, 1989.
4. Charlier R: Antianginal Drugs. Dublin, Heidelberg, New York, Springer Verlag 1971.
5. Massing GK: The clinical pharmacology of antiarrhythmic drugs. In RD Wilkerson (ed): Cardiac Pharmacology. New York, Academic Press, 1981, pp 307–308.
6. Van der Veen FH, Dassen WRM, Havenith MG, et al: In vivo contraction analysis as a measure of canine latissimus dorsi muscle adaptation following chronic electrical stimulation. In RC-J Chiu, I Bourgeois (eds): Transformed Muscle for Cardiac Assist and Repair. Mount Kisco, NY, Futura Publishing Co., 1990, pp 105–115.
7. Havenith MG, Van der Veen FH, Glatz JFC: et al: Monitoring of muscle fiber type of canine latissimus dorsi muscle during chronic electrical stimulation by enzyme and immunohistochemistry. In RC-J Chiu, I Bourgeois (eds): Transformed Muscle

for Cardiac Assist and Repair. Mount Kisco, NY, Futura Publishing Co., 1990, pp 53–61.

8. Magovern GJ, Huckler FR, Park SB, et al: Paced latissimus dorsi used for dynamic cardiomyoplasty of left ventricular aneurysms. Ann Thorac Surg 44:379, 1987.

9. Magovern GJ, Huckler F, Park SB, et al: Paced skeletal muscle for dynamic cardiomyoplasty. Ann Thorac Surg 45:614, 1988.

10. Molteni L, Almada H: Clinical cardiac assist with synchronously stimulated skeletal muscle. J Thorac Cardiovasc Surg 95:940, 1988.

Chapter 20

Skeletal Muscle Ventricle Mechanics: Effects of Passive Stretch

Charles R. Bridges, Jr., Robert L. Hammond,
David R. Anderson, Larry W. Stephenson*

Skeletal muscle ventricles (SMVs) have been constructed and used as cardiac assist devices in vivo as diastolic aortic counterpulsators,[1-5] and more recently, as a replacement for the right ventricle.[6] Spotnitz et al. found that pumping chambers constructed from the canine rectus muscle required preloads of 50 mm Hg or more to generate significant peak pressures.[7] In earlier work in our laboratory, SMVs functioned in mock circulation devices with preloads of 20–40 mm Hg.[8-10] Through application of a theoretical model of the skeletal muscle ventricle,[11,12] we have shown[13] that use of an appropriate SMV chamber size should allow SMVs to be constructed with the appropriate pressure-volume characteristics to perform significant stroke work with preloads in the physiological range. Recently Bridges et al., in our laboratory, confirmed these predictions experimentally, constructing electrically preconditioned SMVs with significant stroke work at preloads in the physiological range of 0–10 mm Hg.[14]

During the vascular delay period, the SMV is similar to a tenotomized muscle, and several investigators[14,15] have shown that some degree of muscle atrophy results. The purpose of the present study was to investigate the effects of passive stretch applied to SMVs during the vascular delay period on the mechanical performance of these SMVs. Sola et al.,[16] Goldspink,[15] and investigators in the field of plastic surgery[17] have evaluated the effects of passive stretch on muscle fibers in a variety of skeletal muscles in the chicken, pig, rabbit, and other species. The application of passive stretch to skeletal muscle consistently results in an increase in muscle mass[15,16] and blood flow.[17] As a result, we devised a simple reliable way of applying stretch to the latissimus dorsi muscle while configured as a skeletal muscle ventricle. The effects of

* Supported by NIH Grant #HLB134778, John Rhea Barton Research Foundation.
From *Cardiomyoplasty* edited by Alain Carpentier, MD, PhD, Juan-Carlos Chachques, MD, and Pierre Grandjean, MS © 1991. Futura Publishing Inc., Mount Kisco, NY.

stretch on passive diastolic and active pressure-volume relations were determined as well as stroke work under a variety of loading conditions and stimulation protocols.

Methods

SMVs were constructed from the left latissimus dorsi muscle in mongrel dogs weighing from 11 to 22 kg. The animals were operated on in accordance with the "Guide for the Care and Use of laboratory Animals" prepared by the National Academy of Sciences (NIH publication No. 85-23, revised 1985). Anesthesia was induced with intravenous thiopental sodium, 2 mg/kg, and maintained with the inhalation of isoflurane. Antibiotic prophylaxis was administered preoperatively, and pain was controlled with parenteral morphine sulphate (0.1 to 0.5 mg/kg). A total of 14 SMVs were constructed in 14 mongrel dogs in each of two groups. In all groups, SMVs were constructed as described below and left undisturbed for 2 to 3 weeks (vascular delay period). Brief definitions of the two groups are: group I (20% stretch, n = 9), group II (no stretch, n = 5).

SMV Construction

In all groups, SMVs were constructed using a technique similar to the one previously developed in our laboratory.[4,5,8,9] SMVs were stimulated via the thoracodorsal nerve. The mandrels used in this study were of two sizes, which volumes of 49 cc (small) and 69 cc (large), significantly larger than the 17 cc mandrels used in some previous studies.[8,9] The large size had a diameter of 3.00 cm at one end, tapered to 2.75 cm at the other end, and a length of 12 cm. The small size had a diameter of 2.5 cm at one end, tapered to 2.3 cm, at the other end, also with a length of 12 cm. In both groups, the ventricles initially were constructed as described above using the small mandrel. In group I (20% stretch), the small mandrel was removed immediately from the SMV after SMV construction and the SMV was stretched by placing the larger mandrel in the same cavity. These SMVs were rested for 2 to 3 weeks prior to the measurements of SMV performance described below.

Mock Circulation System

Stroke work and stroke volume were measured by means of an implantable mock circulation device similar to one described previously.[8,9] We used a recently derived analytical solution for the calculation of stroke work in the mock circulation device.[14]

Measurements

After the animals were anesthetized, the mock circulation device was inserted, and two series of measurements of SMV performance were made—one at 25 Hz, the other at 85 Hz. At each frequency, the previously implanted electrical burst stimulator was programmed to obtain the following settings: duty cycle = 310 ms on, 1.5 sec off; voltage = 4 V (supramaximal in all cases); pulse width = 210 μsec. Stroke work was calculated for SMV contractions with afterloads of 30 mm Hg and preloads of 0 to 25 mm Hg; and with afterloads of 80 mm Hg and preloads of 0 to 55 mm Hg. Isovolumetric SMV pressures, as a function of SMV volume, were obtained for filling volumes of 0 to 40 cc both at the peak of SMV contraction (active) and during the SMV resting phase (passive). The maximum SMV volume at zero filling pressure was recorded as the SMV resting volume, Vo.

Statistics

Comparisons between groups I and II were performed using the two-tailed Student's t-test. Stroke work was compared between the two groups at specified values of the preload pressure.

A polynomial curve-fitting routine was used to summarize the results of the isovolumetric passive and active pressure volume measurements described above. The following procedure was used for each group and for each of the three types of pressure-volume data obtained (passive-diastolic, active–25 Hz, active–85 Hz). The pressure-volume data for all SMVs in each of the two groups for each of the three types of measurements was combined. The resulting six sets of pressure-volume data were individually fitted to quadratic equations relating the pressure (y), to the volume (x). The resulting curves are plotted in Figures 1 and 2. The curve-fitting procedures and statistical comparisons were performed with the RS/1 statistical package (Bolt Baranek and Newman Inc.) on an IBM personal computer.

Results

There were no significant differences between the two groups with respect to dog weight: group I, 15.4 ± 1.5 kg vs. group II, 14.9 ± 1.6 kg. The SMV resting volume, Vo, was significantly higher for group I, 23.6 ± 3.8 cc, than for group II, 10.8 ± 4.0 cc, p <0.05.

Typical pressure tracings from an SMV connected to the mock circulation device are shown in Figure 3. SMV stroke work is plotted as a function of the preload pressure for SMVs of groups I and II in Figure 4. At an afterload of 30 mm Hg and with an 85-Hz burst stimulation frequency, the SMVs that underwent a 20% stretch (group I) developed greater stroke work for a given preload than those without stretch (group II) (Fig. 4B). At an afterload of 30 mm Hg, preload of 10 mm Hg, and an 85-Hz burst stimulation frequency, the stroke work of SMVs in group I averaged 1.1×10^6 ergs; and in group II it averaged 0.77×10^6 ergs.

In contrast, at an afterload of 80 mm Hg and a 25-Hz burst frequency, those SMVs that did *not* undergo stretch (group II) developed greater stroke work (0.86×10^6 ergs at preload = 15 mm Hg) (Fig. 4C). Similarly, with an

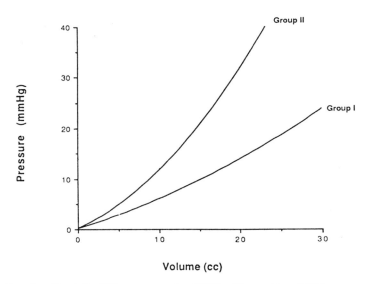

Figure 1. *Passive diastolic filling curves for SMVs. The resting SMV pressure is plotted as a function of volume. At a volume equal to zero on the x axis, the actual volume of fluid within the skeletal muscle ventricle (SMV) is the SMV resting volume (Vo). Therefore, all SMVs are defined to have a resting pressure of zero at volume equal to zero on this graph. Passive diastolic filling curves are shown for group I (20% stretch applied to the SMV at the time of SMV construction) and group II (no stretch applied).*

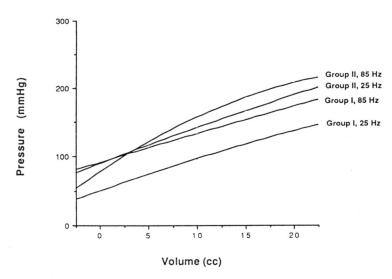

Figure 2. *Active (peak isovolumetric) pressure-volume curves for SMVs. At a volume equal to zero on the x axis, the actual volume of fluid within the skeletal muscle ventricle (SMV) is the SMV resting volume (Vo). Active pressure-volume curves at 25 Hz and 85 Hz are shown for group I (20% stretch applied to the SMV at the time of SMV construction) and group II (no stretch applied).*

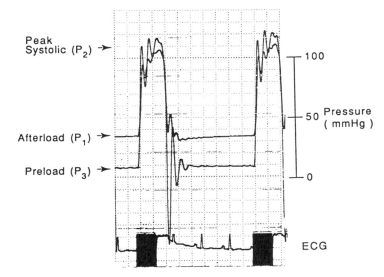

Figure 3. *Typical pressure tracing obtained during mechanical testing of a skeletal muscle ventricle (SMV). At end-diastole, the preload pressure (P_3) is 10 mm Hg and the afterload pressure (P_1) is 30 mm Hg. During systole, the SMV generates a peak pressure (P_2) of approximately 115 mm Hg. Given the three pressures, P_1, P_2, and P_3, the stroke work is calculated as described previously.[14] The electrocardiogram, obtained simultaneously, also is depicted. The superimposed burst pattern corresponds to stimulation of the SMV at 85 Hz.*

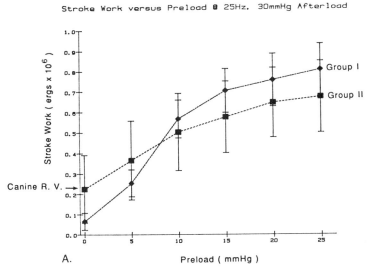

Figure 4. *Stoke work of SMVs. Stroke work as a function of preload is shown for SMVs that were rested for 2 to 3 weeks (vascular delay period) after SMV construction. These SMVs were then subjected to mechanical testing. Group I SMVs had a 20% stretch applied to the muscle fibers at the time of SMV construction, and group II SMVs did not. Arrows associated with "Canine R.V." and "Canine L.V." correspond to the stroke work of the normal canine right and left ventricles, respectively.[4] A. (25 Hz, 30 mm Hg); B. (85 Hz, 30 mm Hg); C. (25 Hz, 80 mm Hg); D. (85 Hz, 80 mm Hg). (A) through (D) correspond to variations in the stimulation frequency and after load pressure of the SMV during mechanical testing with the mock circulation device.*

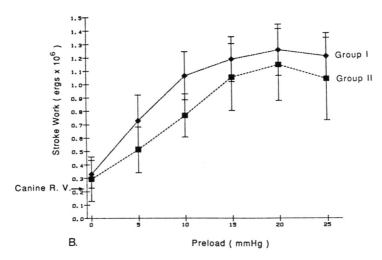

Figure 4B.

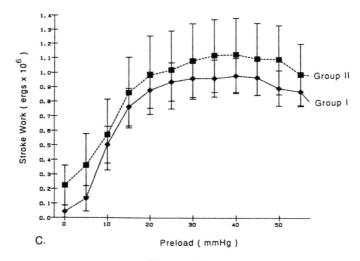

Figure 4C.

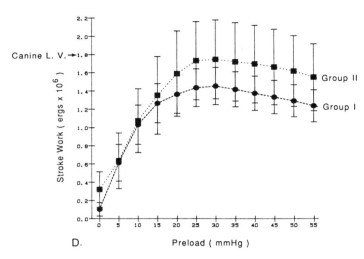

Figure 4D.

85-Hz stimulation frequency and 80-mm Hg afterload, the stroke work for group II was higher than the stroke work for group I (Fig. 4D). At an afterload of 80 mm Hg, preload of 20 mm Hg, and an 85-Hz burst frequency, the stroke work of both group I (1.36×10^6 ergs) and group II (1.59×10^6 ergs) was similar to the stroke work of the normal canine left ventricle,[4] 1.83×10^6 ergs (Fig. 4D). The differences in stroke work between groups I and II were not significant at any preload.

Passive and Active Pressure-Volume Curves

Passive diastolic filling curves, and active pressure-volume curves at 25 Hz and 85 Hz stimulation frequencies for groups I and II are shown in Figures 1 and 2. These curves were derived from the pressure-volume data for each dog in each group. The pressure-volume data from all dogs in any one group was used to fit a quadratic equation to the pressure as a function of volume. For each group, curve fitting was performed for measured passive diastolic pressure (Fig. 1) and peak isovolumetric systolic pressure at 25 Hz and 85 Hz (Fig. 2).

Figure 1 shows that SMVs that were not subjected to stretch were substantially less compliant than SMVs that were subjected to a 20% stretch during the vascular delay period. The slopes of the lines in Figure 2 have been considered as measures of contractility.[18,19] These isovolumetric pressure-volume relationships are analogous to the end-systolic pressure-volume relationships of the left ventricle described by Suga, Sagawa, and others.[18,19] The slope of the curve for group II is higher than the slope of the curve for group I at both 25-Hz and 85-Hz burst frequencies. These slopes are similar in magnitude to the end-systolic elastance of the canine left ventricle.[18,19] Thus the SMVs subjected to a 20% stretch were considerably more compliant, but at the expense of a decrease in contractility. These offsetting influences of passive stretch may explain the lack of a consistent effect on developed stroke work.

Discussion

The results presented here demonstrate that ventricles constructed from skeletal muscle are capable of performing the work necessary to provide significant left ventricular assistance or to effectively supplant right ventricular function, working at the afterloads and preloads of the left and right ventricles, respectively. The SMVs in this study were not electrically preconditioned. Since electrical preconditioning leads to a significant decrease in maximum contractile force,[20] the stroke work achieved here is likely to decrease once these SMVs become converted to a uniform population of type I fatigue-resistant fibers. However, in a companion study we have shown that stroke work comparable to the stroke work achieved here is possible for SMVs that are electrically preconditioned also at physiological preloads and afterloads.[14]

Using our model we were unable to show any consistent effect of stretch on the overall performance of these SMVs. Stretch caused an increase in compliance, which was offset by a decrease in contractility such that there was no consistent effect on developed stroke work. In contrast, we found that stretch did lead to some improvement in stroke work at low preloads in SMVs that were electrically preconditioned.[14] One possible explanation for the results in the present study is that the beneficial effects of passive stretch require more than 2 to 3 weeks to become manifest. For example, in the study by Leighton et al. pig latissimus dorsi muscles underwent passive stretch using tissue expanders for 6 weeks, resulting in a 40%—50% increase in muscle mass and an increase in muscle blood flow.[17]

Since the mandrel used for the SMVs subjected to a 20% stretch was larger than the mandrel used for the control group, we cannot clearly differentiate between the effects of stretch and the effects of larger chamber size. In fact, the alterations in SMV mechanics observed here—increased compliance and decreased end-systolic elastance—associated with passive stretch are precisely the changes that could be predicted to occur from simply increasing the SMV chamber size without stretch.[11,12] To address this issue we are currently enlarging this study to include a group of SMVs constructed with the larger mandrel size without stretch. We will also investigate the performance of this latter group both with and without electrical preconditioning.

Summary

This study indicates that skeletal muscle ventricles can be constructed that have the pressure-volume characteristics appropriate for left- or right-sided cardiac assistance at physiological preloads and afterloads. Passive stretch applied during the vascular delay period leads to inconsistent effects on stroke work developed by SMVs due to a concomitant increase in SMV compliance and a decrease in SMV contractility. The stroke work of these SMVs averaged up to five times the stroke work of the normal canine right ventricle and were similar in magnitude to the stroke work of the canine left ventricle.

References

1. Acker MA, Anderson WA, Hammond RL, et al: Skeletal muscle ventricles in circulation: one to eleven weeks experience. J Thorac Cardiovasc Surg 94:163, 1987.
2. Anderson WA, Bridges CR, Chin AJ, et al: Pneumatic aortic counterpulsator powered by a skeletal muscle ventricle. Surg Forum 39:276, 1988.
3. Chiu RC-J, Walsh GL, Dewar ML, et al: Implantable extra-aortic balloon assist powered by transformed fatigue-resistant skeletal muscle. J Thorac Cardiovasc Surg 94:694, 1987.
4. Mannion JD, Velchik MA, Acker M, et al: Transmural blood flow of multi-layered latissimus dorsi skeletal muscle ventricles during circulatory assistance. Trans Am Soc Artif Intern Organs 32:454, 1986.
5. Mannion JD, Acker MA, Hammond RL, et al: Power output of skeletal muscle ventricles in circulation: short term studies. Circulation 76:155, 1987.
6. Bridges CR, Hammond RL, Dimeo F, et al: Functional right heart replacement with a skeletal muscle ventricle. Circulation (80/Suppl 3):183, 1989.
7. Spotnitz HM, Merker C, Malm JR: Applied physiology of the canine rectus abdominus. Trans Am Soc Artif Intern Organs 20:747, 1974.
8. Acker MA, Hammond RL, Mannion JD, et al: An autologous biologic pump motor. J Thorac Cardiovasc Surg 92:733, 1986.
9. Acker MA, Hammond RL, Mannion JD, et al: Skeletal muscle as a potential power source for a cardiovascular pump: assessment in vivo. Science 236:324, 1987.
10. Anderson WA, Bridges CR, Chin AJ, et al: Trans Am Soc Artif Intern Organs 34:241, 1988.
11. Bridges CR, Stephenson LW: The mechanics of skeletal muscle ventricles: a model based on elasticity theory. In RC-J Chiu, I Bourgeois (eds): Transformed Muscle for Cardiac Assist and Repair. Mount Kisco, NY, Futura Publishing Co, 1989, pp. 255–265.
12. Bridges CR, Anderson JS, Anderson WA, et al: Skeletal muscle ventricles: preliminary results and theoretical design considerations. In B Reichart (ed): Recent Advances in Cardiovascular Surgery. Munich, Verlag RS Schulz, 1989, pp 182–202.
13. Hammond RL, Bridges CR, Dimeo F, et al: Factors in the performance of skeletal muscle ventricles: effects of ventricular chamber size. J Heart Transplant, 9:252, 1990.
14. Bridges CR, Brown WE, Hammond RL, et al: Skeletal muscle ventricles: improved performance at physiological preloads. Surgery 106:275, 1989.
15. Goldspink G: Malleability of the motor system: a comparative approach. J Exp Biol 115:375, 1985.
16. Sola OM, Christensen DL, Martin AW: Hypertrophy and hyperplasia of adult chicken anterior latissimus dorsi muscles following stretch with and without denervation. Exp Neurol 41:76, 1973.
17. Leighton WD, Russell RC, Feller AM, et al: Experimental pretransfer expansion of free-flap donor sites: II. Physiology, histology, and clinical correlation. Plast Reconstr Surg 82:76, 1988.
18. Suga H, Sagawa K: Instantaneous pressure-volume relationships and their ratio in the excised, supported canine left ventricle. Circ Res 35:117, 1974.
19. Igarshi Y, Suga H: Assessment of slope of the end-systolic pressure-volume line of in situ dog heart. Am J Physiol 250:H685, 1986.
20. Mannion JD, Bitto T, Hammond RL, et al: Histochemical and fatigue characteristics of conditioned canine latissimus dorsi muscle. Circ Res 58:298, 1986.

Chapter 21

Skeletal Muscle-Powered Counterpulsation

I. A Critical Overview
Charles R. Bridges, Jr., Robert L. Hammond, David R. Anderson*

II. Adaptation of Stimulation Parameters to Heart Rate
Carlos M. Li, Ray C-J Chiu

III. Chronic Diastolic Counterpulsation†
Roberto Novoa, Delos M. Cosgrove, Lon Castle

A Critical Overview

Presently the only clinical method of skeletal muscle augmentation of the heart is achieved by wrapping muscle around the cardiac ventricles and then stimulating the heart to contract synchronously with cardiac systole.[1-3] Experimentally, skeletal muscle has been used to provide diastolic counterpulsation.[4-7] A number of methods are used that will be described in this chapter. Most of the methods involve wrapping the muscle around the aorta[4] or a relatively small diameter cone or cylinder to create a skeletal muscle ventricle (SMV).[5] The muscle pump then is connected to the circulation and stimulated to contract during cardiac diastole so that the diastolic blood pressure is augmented.

The obvious advantage of the former technique is that sophisticated vascular surgery is not required to use the muscle, blood need not come in contact with the muscle, and the operation can be performed as a single operative

* With the cooperation of A Pochettino, E Hoenhaus, LW Stephenson. Supported by NIH Grant: HL34778.
† With the cooperation of G Jacobs, R Rashidl, C Davies, N Sakakibard.
From *Cardiomyoplasty* edited by Alain Carpentier, MD, PhD, Juan-Carlos Chachques, MD, and Pierre Grandjean, MS © 1991. Futura Publishing Inc., Mount Kisco, NY.

procedure consisting of two parts. The potential disadvantages relate to the different geometric configurations of wrapping the muscle. The ability of the muscle to generate pressure is in general agreement with Laplace's Law, i.e., developed pressure within a cylinder or sphere is inversely proportional to the radius. In the case of the SMV or aortic wrap this radius is much smaller than the ventricular wrap. The ventricular wrap may therefore be less able to generate significant pressures especially in a markedly enlarged heart. When considering very large dilated hearts with biventricular failure it may prove technically difficult to fully wrap these ventricles with the available muscle. Finally and perhaps most important, since skeletal muscle is ordinarily perfused during cardiac systole it may compromise its perfusion to be in a state of tension during this time. This does not suggest that cardiomyoplasty is without value, but that the potential of the SMV concept seems to be a valuable alternative because of specific advantages.

One potential advantage of diastolic skeletal muscle-powered counterpulsation is that the muscle is relaxed during cardiac systole and will be better perfused with blood and therefore less susceptible to fatigue. Furthermore, the ability to generate significant pressure is greater with a small diameter wrap. Four ways in which muscle may be used to augment the diastolic phase of the cardiac cycle are described below along with the advantages and disadvantages of each method.

I. The muscle can be left in situ except for its proximal insertion on the humerus, which is detached and reimplanted on the first or second rib. A space is developed on its deep surface between the muscle and chest wall into which a bladder is inserted. This bladder is linked to the aorta such that contraction of the muscle compresses the bladder that in turn displaces a volume of blood in the aorta. The system may employ a hydraulic or pneumatic drive between the bladder and a displacement chamber (Fig. 1), which is placed in series with the aorta. Alternatively, blood may be allowed to fill the bladder direct. This system avoids extensive dissection and division of collateral blood vessels to the muscle, and the surgery required is technically simple to perform. The efficiency of transfer of longitudinal force developed by the muscle into compression of the bladder is not known, however, but it is likely to be low. Any hydraulic or pneumatic drive system will tend to absorb energy, further reducing efficiency. In addition, because of the ability of gases and fluids to slowly leak through all presently available synthetic materials, the system would need regular "top-ups" to maintain its working capacity. If blood is allowed to directly fill the bladder, thus dispensing with the need for an indirect drive, thrombosis may become a major problem.

II. The muscle may be fully mobilized and wrapped around a bladder connected to the circulation as in (I) (Fig. 2)[6,7]. This is likely to be more efficient in transmitting longitudinal force to compression of the bladder but has the same disadvantages of thrombosis or loss of energy if a hydraulic or pneumatic drive is used.

III. Kantrowitz, a pioneer in this field, wrapped muscle around a mobilized segment of descending thoracic aorta (Fig. 3). This method provides a distinct advantage in that it avoids the need for any kind of hydraulic or pneumatic

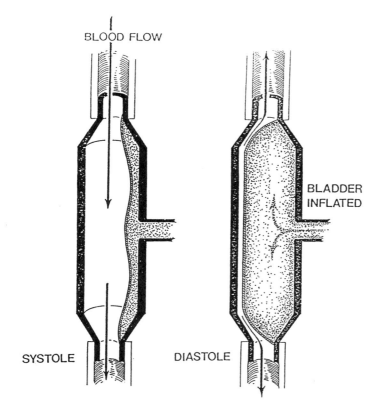

BLOOD FLOW

BLADDER
INFLATED

SYSTOLE   DIASTOLE

Figure 1. *The displacement chamber consists of an outer case with an inner flexible bladder that expands within the casing to displace blood in both directions. Gas or fluid may be used to inflate the bladder.*

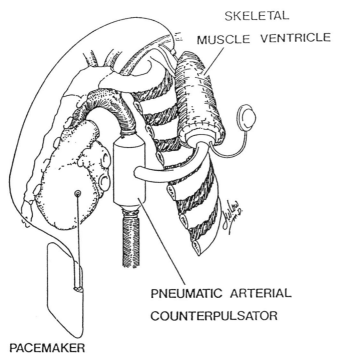

SKELETAL

MUSCLE VENTRICLE

PNEUMATIC ARTERIAL

COUNTERPULSATOR

PACEMAKER

Figure 2. *The muscle has been fully mobilized and wrapped around a bladder that in this case is connected indirectly to the aorta via a displacement chamber. Alternatively blood may enter the bladder direct from the aorta.*

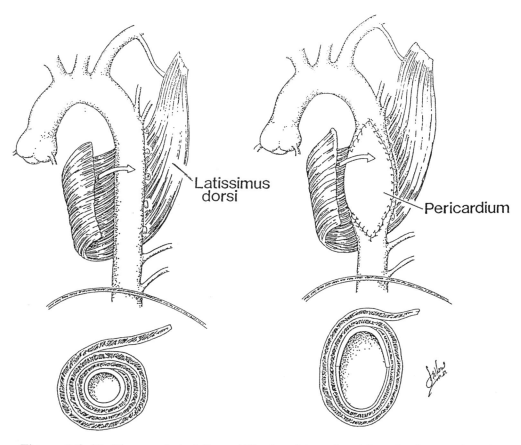

Figure 3 (left). *The muscle is fully mobilized and introduced into the thorax where it is wrapped around the descending aorta after division of a number of intercostal branches.* **Figure 4 (right).** *The aorta is enlarged to increase the volume of blood that is compressed. Pericardium or any flexible material can be used.*

drive while retaining good transfer of longitudinal force into compression. In addition, blood does not come in contact with muscle or any other thrombogenic surface. A potential disadvantage is that mobilization of sufficient aorta may involve division of too many intercostal branches leading to spinal cord ischemia. Moreover, the aorta in patients requiring this kind of treatment may be atheromatous or calcific, and rhythmic compression of such an aorta has obvious potential hazards. Finally, the volume of blood displaced will depend on the volume of aorta encompassed. In some cases this may be quite small given the muscle width and aortic diameter. A possible solution to the latter point is to enlarge the aorta by incorporating a patch into the wall (Fig. 4) in order to create an aneurysm. While such a procedure may be acceptable in an experimental model it is an unattractive clinical alternative.

IV. Instead of wrapping the aorta, the mobilized muscle can be wrapped around a Teflon mandrel of predetermined volume and dimensions. After a

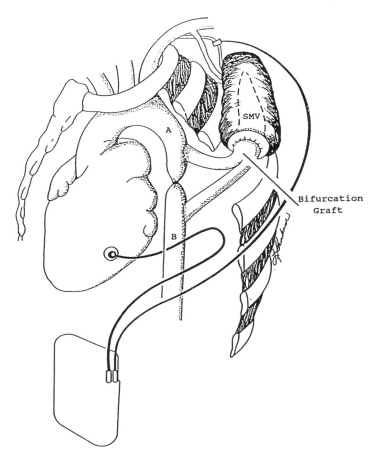

Figure 5. *The skeletal muscle ventricle (SMV) is connected directly to the descending aorta using a Gore-Tex® bifurcation graft. The graft enters the chest through the bed of the fourth rib which has been resected. At operation, ultrasonic flow probes are placed around the aorta at A and B and the flow dynamics generated by the contracting SMV analyzed. – – – = the autogenous lining of the SMV.*

delay period of approximately 4 weeks, the Teflon is removed leaving a cavity in the muscle wrap referred to as a skeletal muscle ventricle (SMV). This delay period allows adhesions to form between the two layers of muscle. It has been shown that there is recovery of exercise-induced blood flow to the muscle as compared to immediately after surgical mobilization.[8] The resulting cavity then is anastomosed to the descending aorta such that blood enters the cavity and on contraction is ejected back into the circulation via either the same conduit (Fig. 2) or a separate conduit from the same (Fig. 5) or opposite end of the SMV (Fig. 6). The advantage here is that there is efficient transfer of muscle energy to the circulation. The disadvantage to date has been the tendency for thrombus formation within the SMV cavity and subsequent throm-

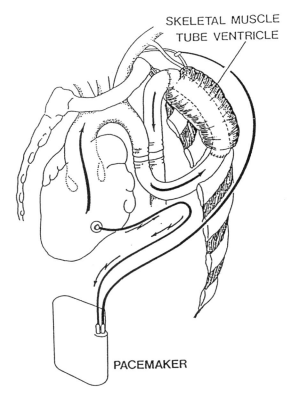

Figure 6. *This configuration allows blood to enter the SMV at one end and exit the other. This configuration also reduces the tendancy to stasis (ref. 5).*

boembolism even when the cavity has been lined with a relatively low thrombogenic material such as polytetrafluoroethelene (PTFE).[5]

In a series of experiments where SMVs were connected to a totally implantable mock circulation device, SMVs constructed as described in (IV) were shown to be capable of significant, continuous, and chronic work in an awake animal.[9] No tubes or wires crossed the skin except during measurements. The system allowed control of preload and afterload as well as measurement of pressure and flow produced, while avoiding the problems of thrombosis and synchronous burst stimulation that might have occurred had the SMVs been connected to the circulation. SMVs, which had been electrically preconditioned, pumped continuously against a pressure of 80 mm Hg with a preload of 40 mm Hg at a rate of 54 contractions per minute for up to 9 weeks. After 2 weeks of continuous pumping, the systolic pressure generated by the SMVs was 104 $+/-1$ mm Hg and fluid displacement was 206 $+/-$ 16 mL/min.

In a subsequent experiment,[10] we found that electrical preconditioning was not absolutely necessary for SMVs to perform sustained work in the dog. SMVs were constructed and allowed a period of vascular delay only. After 2 weeks of pumping into the mock circulation, SMVs without electrical preconditioning generated stroke work of 0.04 +/− 0.014J at standard settings of 25-Hz burst frequency, preload 40 mm Hg and afterload 80 mm Hg. This represents about 25% of the stroke work of the left ventricle in the dog and almost equals the stroke work of the right ventricle. Although there was some decrease in pressure and flow over a period of 1 month, the end result was similar with or without electrical preconditioning.

The SMVs pumped continuously against a mock circulation system at preloads of 40 mm Hg, but significant stroke work was also produced at physiological preloads, which suggested that it should be possible to construct SMVs with a compliance similar to that of the left ventricle. Later, SMVs were constructed, allowing a vascular recovery period but no electrical preconditioning. They were connected to the aorta using a flow-through technique[5] and stimulated to contract during cardiac diastole. Two dogs survived for 5 and 11 weeks, respectively, with the SMV pumping continuously as a diastolic counterpulsator. During this period there was significant and sustained augmentation of the diastolic blood pressure. Death was due to renal failure secondary to repeated thromboemboli from the SMV. The SMVs were lined with PTFE.

At this stage of development, option (IV) probably offers the most efficient means of using skeletal muscle energy to provide aortic diastolic counterpulsation. Therefore, our aim is to develop a nonthrombogenic lining for these SMVs. The first possibility is to use a prosthetic material such as PTFE. This has not, however, been totally successful in controlling thromboembolism. Moreover, prosthetic materials have potential drawbacks such as risk of infection and fibrous encapsulation that might eventually lead to a reduction in SMV compliance. Due to constant flexing material fatigue also is a problem. Polyurethane, however, shows remarkable resistance to fatigue in in vitro studies. Another disadvantage is that prosthetic materials offer no potential for growth therefore limiting the possible usefulness of this kind of therapy in pediatric patients.

The solution may be to line the ventricles with a living tissue capable of regeneration and repair. Such tissue should be autogenously derived to avoid immune problems. Possibilities include pericardium, pleura, and vascular tissue.

A series of experiments have been conducted to evaluate the thrombogenicity of various biological linings for SMVs. Skeletal muscle ventricles were constructed in dogs according to the standard method used in this laboratory. The muscle was mobilized on its neurovascular pedicle through a long flank incision. Two or three large collateral vessels that emerge from the fifth and sixth intercostal spaces were preserved as they do not interfere with the next stage which is to wrap the muscle in a double layer around a tapering Teflon mandrel of predetermined dimensions. A specially modified electrode was placed carefully on the thoracodorsal nerve and tunneled through to the rectus sheath. The SMVs were constructed with three different linings: either the natural fibrous reaction induced by the Teflon mandrel during the 3- to 4-week vascular recovery period (this fibrous lining serves as a control) or autogeneously derived pericardium or pleura. After a vascular delay period of 4 weeks without electrical preconditioning, a second operation was performed to remove the Teflon mandrel and to anatomose the SMV to the descending thoracic aorta using a bifurcation graft. The proximal end of the graft was connected to the SMV, and each limb was connected separately to the aorta. The aorta was then ligated between the limbs of the graft such that there would be obligatory blood flow through the SMV (Fig. 5).

A Gore-Tex® PTFE graft was chosen because of the low thrombogenicity of this material in the dog and particularly because the alignment of the two limbs somewhat mimics the configuration of the inflow and outflow portions of the left ventricle. It was hoped that by pointing so directly at the apex of the SMV the inflow limb would provide effective washing of that region and prevent thrombosis due to stasis. At this stage, six dogs survive with SMVs pumping continuously in circulation. Two dogs with pleural linings are entirely free of thrombosis as confirmed by ultrasound after 12 and 3 weeks. Both show excellent augmentation of the diastolic blood pressure (Fig. 7). This augmented pressure is due to increased blood flow confirmed by intraoperative ultrasonic flow probes around the aorta and postoperative doppler interrogation of the femoral artery (Fig. 8). Two others with pleural linings have organizing thrombus in the distal third of the cavity. Two with pericardial linings currently are free of thrombus at 1 and 2 weeks, respectively. Weekly blood tests to assess renal function show no evidence of impairment, which has been seen due to repeated embolization.[5] All control SMVs have developed thrombus at an early stage.

The only nonthrombogenic lining known is living vascular endothelium. If this can be grown in the SMV, thrombosis should not be a problem. Two possibilities exist: to use a blood vessel to line the cavity or to seed the cavity with endothelial cells. Our early attempts with blood vessels have been hampered by insufficient readily available autogenous vessel to provide 100% lining of the SMV cavity. The IVC is a possibility but harvesting would involve extensive surgery.

Vascular endothelial cell-seeding for lining prostheses is an exciting possibility currently attracting a lot of attention in vascular surgery. If endothelial cells can be made to adhere and proliferate on the fibrous base created by the Teflon mandrel, a solution to the problem of thrombosis may be provided. Finally, our experimental work has been conducted in the dog and the results obtained may not necessarily apply to humans. The dog is a notoriously thrombogenic animal compared to a human, and the only anticoagulant used in these experiments was aspirin. Systemic heparin was not employed at operation. With the use of heparin and/or coumarin, it may be possible to effectively control thrombosis in humans.

Another consideration concerns the correct timing of stimulation of the SMV. Intra-aortic balloon pumping (IABP), an effective method for diastolic augmentation of a failing left ventricle achieves its effect by a combination of two actions: (1) diastolic pumping with pressure augmentation and (2) left ventricular afterload reduction. As a result, timing of balloon inflation and deflation is critical in order to optimize the benefit and prevent the IABP from working against the heart. By placing ultrasonic flow probes around the aorta just proximal and just distal to the points of attachment of the two limbs of

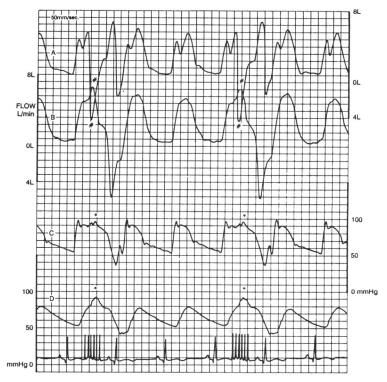

Figure 7. *Examples of ultrasonic flow and pressure tracings obtained immediately after connection of the SMV to the circulation. "A" is the flow trace at position "A" (Fig. 5). Contraction of the SMV induces retrograde flow in the distal aortic arch (#). "B" represents the flow trace recorded at position "B" (Fig. 5). Contraction induces a surge in forward flow (#). Coincident with SMV contraction there is an increase in carotid (C) and femoral (D) diastolic blood pressure (*). The ECG shows the superimposed stimulation burst, which in this case is at 25 Hz frequency, R-wave delay of 225 ms, and duration of 240 ms.*

the bifurcation graft, we have observed a similar critical relationship between the timing of the SMV contraction and cardiac systole. Examples of different flow patterns obtained are shown in Figure 9. Example (A) demonstrates the effect of correct timing. There is good diastolic augmentation, and since the impulse burst terminates just before the next R wave there is good afterload reduction as the SMV relaxes. The Doppler flow tracing illustrates that the subsequent cardiac systole has a greatly increased velocity and volume when compared to a normal beat. In (B) there is a significant gap between the end of the impulse burst and the next cardiac systole. As a result, the subsequent systole is nonaugmented when compared to a beat not following contraction of the SMV. In other words, there is no afterload reduction. In example (C) the impulse burst extends beyond the next R wave such that the SMV is contracting against the left ventricle. These recordings are taken in the context

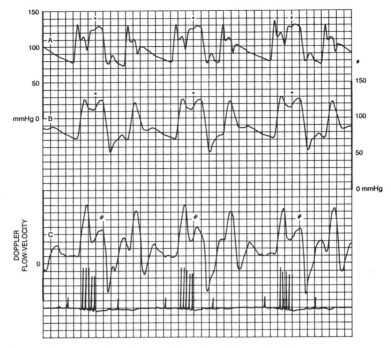

Figure 8. *Tracings recorded from a dog after 12 weeks of continuous pumping with configuration as in Fig. 5. "A" is the brachial artery pressure; "B" is the femoral artery pressure. (*) represents the diastolic pressure augmentation with the SMV contracting with every other heart beat. "C" is the Doppler flow trace recorded from the femoral artery using a transcutaneous 8.4 MHz probe placed at an angle of less than 45° to the femoral artery. (#) shows the increase in flow velocity as the SMV contracts. Stimulation frequency 25 Hz, R-wave delay 200 ms, burst duration 185 ms, amplitude 2.5 V.*

of a normal heart but a situation such as (C) might not be tolerated by a failing heart.

These examples were obtained using the currently available Cardiomyostimulator™ Pulse Train Generator (Medtronic Model SP1005). This stimulator only allows programming of the R-wave delay and burst duration. As a result, with a fluctuating heart rate the relative relationship of the impulse burst to the next R wave will vary. This problem is now being addressed with a new stimulator that will allow the timing of the impulse burst to maintain a constant relationship within the R-R interval.

At this stage there is not sufficient evidence to justify clinical application of skeletal muscle ventricles as diastolic counterpulsators. Nevertheless, the results obtained thus far are encouraging and clearly indicate that skeletal muscle is capable of adapting to chronic usage without fatiguing to a point of uselessness. Since it has been shown that SMVs can perform useful work at physiological preloads, there is the possibility that a congenitally deficient or irreversibly damage right ventricle could be replaced. Cardiomyoplasty does

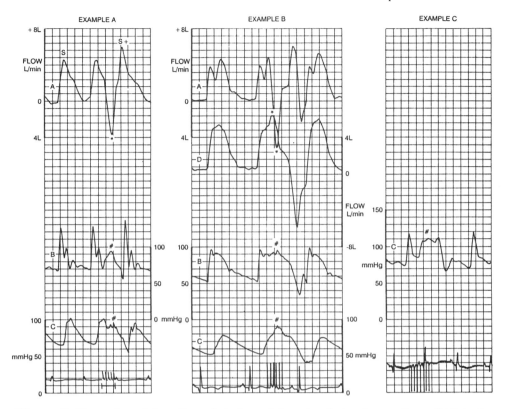

Figure 9. *Examples of the effect of timing of the stimulation burst. Trace "A" is the ultrasonic flow recorded just distal to the aortic arch but proximal to the bifurcation graft (see Fig. 5). "B" is the carotid artery pressure. "C" is the femoral artery pressure. "D" is the flow recorded just distal to the bifurcation graft. In example A "S" represents the flow in a normal systole. "S+" is the flow following SMV contraction. The velocity and volume are both increased. In example B, the SMV contraction terminates too soon such that there is no increase in the velocity or volume of the next systole. In example C, the SMV contraction overruns the next systole and from the pressure trace it can be seen to encroach on the pressure wave. No flows are available here as this recording was obtained several days after surgery.*

not appear to have this potential. Presently, work output is insufficient for total replacement of the left ventricle but good assist can be achieved.

Several issues remain to be resolved. The problem of thrombosis has been discussed. There is also the question of what will happen to a muscle ventricle subjected to systemic pressures on a long-term basis. The best method of construction of an SMV has yet to be decided. Better SMV design or configuration may allow for increased work output approaching that of the left ventricle.

II. Adaptation of Stimulation Parameters to Heart Rate

It is now feasible to use autologous skeletal muscle as a biomechanical assist of the heart. After extensive laboratory investigations, dynamic cardiomyoplasty has reached the clinical trial phase of evaluation.[3,11,12] Several institutions presently are involved in determining the efficacy of cardiomyoplasty. However, the best method of applying the potential energy source in skeletal muscle remains an issue. The purpose of this chapter is to briefly review the undergoing progress in alternative forms of muscle-powered assist.

Kantrowitz in 1959 was one of the first to use skeletal muscle for cardiac assist.[4] He accomplished this by wrapping a portion of the diaphragm around the thoracic aorta and stimulating it to contract during diastole for counterpulsation. With this method, he was able to achieve a 27% increase in mean arterial pressure. Other investigators followed with similar concepts of muscle-powered assist devices, although, with limited success.[13-15] The problem of muscle fatigue remained a major obstacle that discouraged further investigation in this area. In the early 1980s, introduction of the principle of skeletal muscle transformation helped revitalize the field of biomechanical assist.[16] It is now believed that skeletal muscle can be made fatigue resistant through chronic stimulation and used for continuous cardiac assist.

In 1985, Neilson et al. used an extra-aortic balloon pump driven by skeletal muscle to provide counterpulsation assist.[17] In this system, a vascular graft was anastomosed to the thoracic aorta and connected to a polyurethane bulb. The bulb was then brought underneath the muscle where it would be compressed during diastole. Significant counterpulsation was produced by this action. We believe this setup offers several advantages over cardiomyoplasty. First, it takes advantage of systolic pressures to preload the muscle. It has been demonstrated that skeletal muscle requires high preloads of approximately 30–40 mm Hg to function optimally. Such high filling pressures are not feasible with dynamic cardiomyoplasty. Second, dissection of the muscle is minimized since there is no need to mobilize it for wrapping around the heart. This helps preserve collateral circulation which plays an important role in preventing muscle fatigue. Finally, there is the possibility of detrimental paradoxical motion for every unassisted beat in cardiomyoplasty, while in a counterpulsation system no harm results in unassisted beats. This would allow more flexibility when progressively training the muscle where a gradual increase in workload can be achieved.

Based on the success of Neilson's work, we have continued to investigate this area of counterpulsation assist. In 1987 we duplicated the same effective counterpulsation using transformed fatigue-resistant muscle.[7] At that time, it became clear that design changes were needed for the extra-aortic pump. Due to the end-bud design of the pump, significant clotting occurred from the blood stasis. In 1988 Kochamba et al. introduced a "dual-chambered" extra-aortic counterpulsation pump concept for use with skeletal muscle power.[6] The pump is anastomosed in parallel to the thoracic aorta. This provides for a continuous through flow of blood, which prevents stasis and clotting. Counterpulsation is provided by collapse of a flexible polyurethane membrane within the pump by muscle contraction on a pneumatic bulb (Fig. 10). To use this pump in a chronic model, a special pulse generator was developed for stimulating the muscle.

Timing must be continuously adjusted according to heart rate if effective

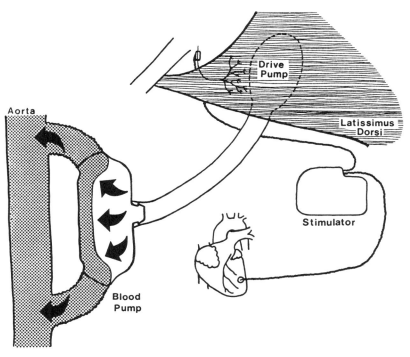

Figure 10. *Schematic representation of system using dual-chambered counterpulsation pump. The pump is anastomosed in parallel to the descending aorta. Contraction of the muscle on the drive bulb during diastole results in collapse of a flexible membrane, effecting counterpulsation assist. (Reprinted with permission from Li et al: Trans Am Soc Artif Int Organs 35, 1989.)*

counterpulsation is to be maintained. Medtronic Inc. recently developed an implantable muscle stimulator that delivers pulse bursts synchronized to the R wave of the ECG.[18] A built-in microprocessor senses the R-R intervals and tailors the delay period and burst duration accordingly. As a result, varying heart rate is tracked by R-R interval changes, and automatic adjustments are made to maintain optimal timing for counterpulsation. Programming of the stimulator is accomplished with personal computer software and is transmitted via telemetry. An additional feature of the stimulator is its ability to detect arrhythmias and to shut down temporarily when such events occur.

Using the available equipment, we have developed an implantable counterpulsation assist system (ICAS). The dual-chambered pump and the rate-responsive stimulator were combined in an animal model to provide effective counterpulsation. Counterpulsation equivalent to the intra-aortic balloon was achieved with the ICAS, where diastolic pressure augmentation of 70%, and systolic unloading of 11% from baseline were easily demonstrated. When heart rate was varied, the system readjusted the timing thus maintaining effective counterpulsation (Fig. 11). Additional features of the ICAS include the ability to detect and shut down during arrhythmias and compatibility with intra-

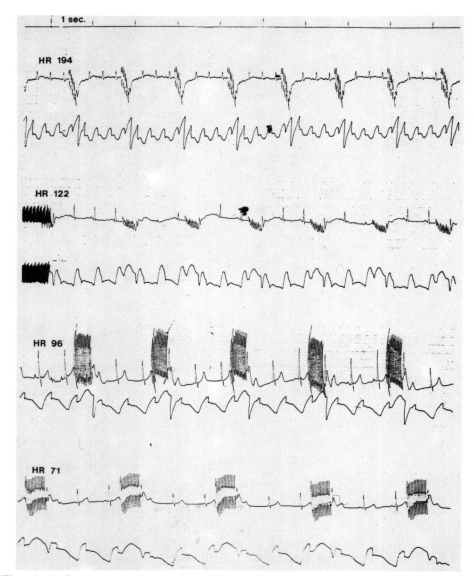

Figure 11. *Pressure tracings at four different heart rates. As heart rate changes, there are automatic adjustments in timing of the assist, and effective counterpulsation is maintained. (Reprinted with permission from Li et al: Trans Am Soc Artif Int Organs 35, 1989.)*

aortic balloon pump consoles which act as a backup power source. Chronic studies of the ICAS are continuing in an effort to further evaluate and refine the system.

Currently, it appears unlikely that muscle-powered devices will be able to assume the full workload of the left ventricle. Most studies that have measured the power output of such devices achieve between 20%–60% of the LV output. However, the power output is highly dependent upon the efficiency and design of the system. It has been shown that skeletal muscle can generate up to 2.4 kg/cm^2 active tension, while myocardium generates 0.6 kg/cm^2 active tension.[19] Theoretically, a large muscle like the latissimus dorsi should be capable of completely supporting the heart if an efficient device could be designed. Much work remains to be done in this area of muscle-powered assist. At this time, the main goal for the ICAS and other similar systems is to support failing hearts with some residual function. Recent reports of patients on chronic intra-aortic balloon support demonstrate the need for such devices. The rapid successful transition from laboratory to clinical trials of dynamic cardiomyoplasty reflects the rapid advances in the field of biomechanical assist. Hopefully, development of muscle-powered counterpulsation systems will progress similarly.

III. Chronic Diastolic Counterpulsation

The use of skeletal muscle for cardiac assistance has generated a great deal of interest as a possible alternative in the treatment of congestive heart failure. Although this interest dates back several decades, the initial results were hindered by the fatigability of skeletal muscle when stimulated to perform continuous work.[4,20] Subsequent investigations by Stephenson's group demonstrated that skeletal muscle could be rendered fatigue resistant following a period of electrical conditioning.[21,22]

Research on skeletal muscle for cardiac assistance has been directed along two major avenues: (1) dynamic cardiomyoplasty where the muscle is wrapped directly around the ventricle and (2) diastolic counterpulsation, an assist modality that has been helpful in a large number of patients with acute heart failure[23] and seems to be of benefit in selected long-term patients.[24] Although cardiomyoplasty is currently undergoing clinical trials with encouraging results,[3,11] experiments in counterpulsation have been fraught with major difficulties such as thromboembolism[5] and obtaining appropriate synchronization of the muscle contraction to the cardiac cycle.[25] The purpose of this research was to develop an experimental model for assessing the requirements of muscle-assisted counterpulsation.

Material and Methods

Following initial viability experiments to establish a feasible experimental model, five adult mongrel dogs were anesthetized with pentobarbital 30 mg/kg. The left latissimus dorsi was dissected through a longitudinal incision parallel to the free border. The muscle was detached from its origin and insertion and the collateral blood supply ligated and divided except for a major collateral in the region of the fourth intercostal space. A bipolar cuff electrode was placed around the thoracodorsal nerve and connected to an Itrel™ pacemaker (Medtronic, Inc.). Strong muscle contractions could be elicited with

		Time On	Time Off	
Postop Week	Rate (bpm)	(sec)	(sec)	On/Off Ratio
0–4	0	–	–	–
5–8	54	310	810	1:2.6
9	60	250	750	1:3
10	64	250	690	1:2.8
11	87	190	500	1:2.6

Table 1
Conditioning Protocol

pulse bursts of 0.5 V and a pulse width of 210 μsec. The muscle was then wrapped around a 30-cc mandrel that was fixed to the chest wall in the area of the third intercostal space. The incision was closed and the animals allowed to recover.

After a 3- to 4-week period of vascular delay to allow the muscle to recover from the lost collateral blood supply, muscle conditioning was started using the protocol outlined in Table 1. The voltage and pulse width were adjusted as needed to produce a strong contraction. Following 12 weeks of conditioning, the dogs were anesthetized and the mandrel was excised and replaced with a 42-cc elliptical pericardial reservoir. This reservoir was connected to the circulation by means of 10-mm vascular grafts (Gore-tex) anastomosed to the aorta end to side. The aorta was then ligated between the two anastomoses to increase blood flow through the pericardial bladder and hence reduce stagnation (Fig. 12). A myocardial sensing lead (Medtronic Model 6917T) was placed in the left ventricle and connected to the sensing port of the pacemaker system. The leads from the cuff electrode were detached from the Itrel™ pacemaker (Medtronic, Inc.) and connected to the muscle channel of the Cardiomyostimulator™ Pulse Train Generator (Medtronic Model SP1005). The pacemaker was programmed to stimulate the muscle every other heart beat (mode II) and ECG and arterial pressures were recorded on a Hewlett-Packard chart recorder.

Results

Initial results showed that with a stimulation delay of 250 ms, the pressure wave generated by the muscle contraction occurred before the dicrotic notch thus increasing left ventricular impedance (Fig. 13). Analysis of electrocardiograms and pressure tracings revealed that over a range of 60 to 120 bpm, the interval from the QRS to the dicrotic notch ranged from 380 to 430 ms, which was beyond the range provided by the Cardiomyostimulator™ Pulse Train Generator.

A pacemaker system was developed from currently available hardware capable of providing delays from 8 to 500 ms.[10] It consisted of connecting a

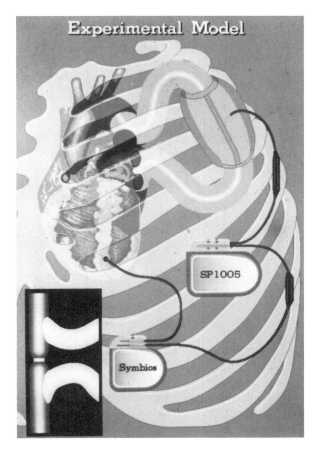

Figure 12. *Pericardial reservoir surrounded by conditioned latissimus dorsi muscle tube.*

Symbios™ DDD pacemaker (Medtronic, Inc.) in series with a Cardiomyostimulator™ Pulse Train Generator using a voltage divider. Bench tests demonstrated that 1:1 stimulation could be maintained up to 100 bpm. Above this value, the pacemaker would cause a Wenckebach phenomenon and the muscle channel would emit a series of pulses every other beat. Other stimulation protocols could be achieved by changing the refractory periods of both the SP1005 and the Symbios™ pacemakers; however, certain combinations resulted in poor synchronization of the muscle contraction to the cardiac cycle.

The optimal stimulation delay was determined by observing the hemodynamics resulting from delays of 250, 300, 350, and 400 ms (Fig 14). Surprisingly, the optimal delay was 350 ms and not the expected 400 ms. Further analysis of these tracings explained the reason for this finding: the skeletal muscle tube required 30 to 60 ms before it could generate sufficient tension to overcome the systemic pressure at the dicrotic notch (Fig. 15).

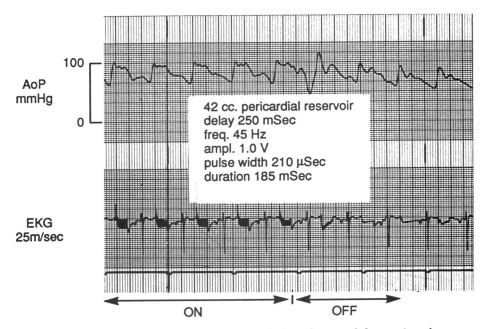

Figure 13. *Counterpulsation occurring before closure of the aortic valve.*

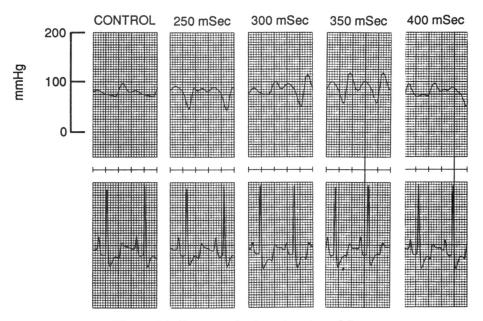

Figure 14. *Counterpulsation at various delays.*

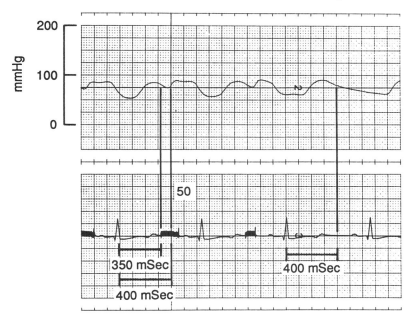

Figure 15. *Pressure-synchronization delay relationship.*

The hemodynamic effects of counterpulsation were analyzed by comparing the systolic, peak diastolic, and end-diastolic pressures of ten beats with and without assistance. Each dog served as its own control and the results were evaluated using paired *t*-tests. There was no significant difference in the systolic pressures with and without assistance (Fig. 16). The assisted or augmented diastolic pressure was higher in all animals but significantly so in four out of five. The augmented diastolic pressure was not significantly different from the systolic pressures. The assisted end-diastolic pressure, which is related to systolic unloading of the ventricle, was lower in all dogs but significant in only three animals. Diastolic augmentation increased by an average of 19% and systolic unloading averaged 23%.

The effect of stimulation delay on the systemic pressure is shown in Figure 17. The pacemakers were programmed to stimulate the muscle tube at 250, 325, 350, and 400 ms after sensing the R wave. The best augmentation and unloading were obtained with a delay of 350 ms, although there was very little difference between 350 and 325 ms.

One dog was electively sacrificed at 1½ weeks because of high thresholds required for muscle stimulation. The pericardial sac was lined with a thin layer of fibrin and was free of clots except for a small area at the suture lines. To a large extent, the latissimus dorsi muscle was replaced by fibrosis, most likely related to vascular compromise of the pedicle. The remaining four dogs died abruptly at 5 to 6 weeks after the second procedure. Autopsy findings showed the cause of death to be secondary to massive thromboembolism to the abdominal aorta. The clots were well formed and appeared to have originated

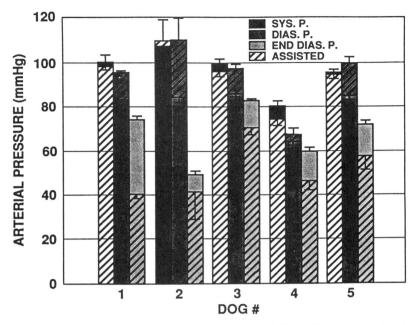

Figure 16. *Hemodynamic effects of muscle-powered diastolic counterpulsation.*

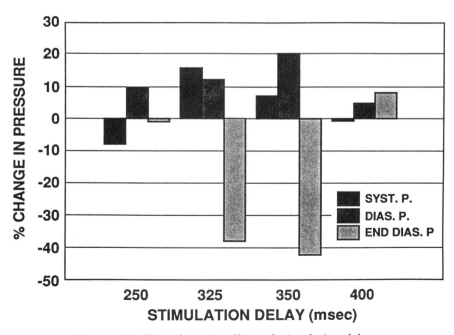

Figure 17. *Hemodynamic effects of stimulation delays.*

in the pericardial reservoir, which at this time was lined with a layer of clots. On gross examination, the muscle tubes had a variable amount of fibrosis.

Discussion

The use of skeletal muscle to produce counterpulsation has evolved for a variety of reasons. Principally, the experimental evidence indicates that the working capacity of skeletal muscle ventricles against systemic afterloads is marginal and also preload-dependent. In addition, the excellent results of intra-aortic balloon pumping in the clinical setting, the absence of valves, and the possibility of an endogenously reliable and inexpensive power source have contributed to the interest in muscle-powered counterpulsation devices. Mannion and coworkers[21,22] have demonstrated that the power output of ventricles fashioned from conditioned canine latissimus dorsi muscle is intermediate between that of the right and left ventricles. Diastolic counterpulsation has been useful clinically in patients with heart failure,[23] and its power requirements are a fraction of that needed for parallel left ventricular assistance. Spotnitz et al.[14] demonstrated that pouches constructed of skeletal muscle behave in a manner reminiscent of the Frank-Starling law; however, the optimal preload pressure was above 50 mm Hg, which is in the same range as the systemic diastolic pressure.

Using a variety of animal models, several groups have documented that skeletal muscle can generate sufficient tension for counterpulsation.[6,7,21,22] Acker et al.[9] employed an implantable mock circulation system to determine the long-term ability of trained muscle to sustain continuous work. They were able to show that the canine latissimus dorsi muscle was able to generate a stroke work of 1.2×10^3 ergs for periods ranging from 8 to 63 days. Pressures up to 243 mm Hg were generated without evidence of muscle fatigue. Kochamba and colleagues,[6] using a a two-chamber device connected to the aorta found that the in situ latissimus dorsi muscle could generate enough force to produce counterpulsation, thus obviating the need for a prolonged vascular delay that is necessary when the muscle is dissected completely.[23]

Although the use of muscle power for circulatory assistance is clearly viable, delivering this energy into the circulation has been hindered by the occurrence of thromboembolism. All long-term attempts, including the present one, have resulted in fatalities secondary to thromboembolism. In an attempt to avoid foreign material in contact with the blood, some investigators have wrapped the muscle around the aorta with encouraging short-term results as evidence from the works of Chachques and Pattison in this volume. Although attractive for its simplicity and blood compatibility aspects, possible drawbacks are: the risk of paraplegia from ligation of intercostal vessels, the inability to displace enough volume to achieve significant assistance, the possibility of arterial emboli arising from compression of an atherosclerotic aorta, and damage to the vessel wall.

Another major concern in counterpulsation is the special stimulation protocols required to produce satisfactory synchronization with the cardiac cycle.

Current intra-aortic balloon pumps have complex algorithms that are capable of determining the appropriate inflation and deflation of the balloon.[26] Even with these devices, supervision by trained personnel is required to achieve optimal hemodynamic assistance. In our initial work,[25] we demonstrated that delays of 350 ms were needed to produce well-timed counterpulsation. In addition, it is clear that the delay and duration necessary for diastolic counterpulsation will depend on the step response rate of the system, i.e., muscle pumps with fast responses will need longer delays than slower responding configurations. Although the interval from the QRS to dicrotic notch decreases slightly with increasing heart rates, the length of diastole is shortened to a even greater degree. Thus, systems based on fixed or percent delays are not likely to be useful except for cases with fixed heart rates, i.e., pacemaker-dependent patients.

Yet another problem in muscle-assisted counterpulsation is the time period necessary for vascular delay and electrical conditioning. During the 8–12 weeks when these processes are taking place, the patient would be receiving suboptimal hemodynamic support. Even after this time interval, disastrous consequences would result should the muscle fail due to trauma to its nerve, inadequate blood supply, or general inability to meet the demands imposed upon it. Clearly, a substitute power source would be needed during times of marginal power output.

Conclusions

Muscle-assisted diastolic counterpulsation is an area of promising research in the field of circulatory assistance. Although major problems such as thromboembolism and stimulation protocols need to be solved, the experimental evidence thus far suggests that this form of assistance has potential application in the treatment of patients with refractory congestive heart failure.

References

1. Carpentier A, Chachques JC: Myocardial substitution with a stimulated skeletal muscle: first successful clinical case. Lancet i:1267, 1985.
2. Magovern GJ, Park SB, Magovern GJ Jr, et al: Latissimus dorsi as a functioning synchronously paced muscle component in the repair of a left ventricular aneurysm. Ann Thorac Surg 41:116, 1986.
3. Molteni L, Almada H, Ferreira R: Synchronously stimulated skeletal muscle graft for left ventricular assistance. Case report. J Thorac Cardiovasc Surg 97:439, 1989.
4. Kantrowitz A, McKinnon WMP: The experimental use of the diaphragm as an auxiliary myocardium. Surg Forum 9:266, 1959.
5. Acker MA, Anderson WA, Hammond RL, et al: Skeletal muscle ventricles in circulation. One to eleven weeks' experience. J Thorac Cardiovasc Surg 94:163, 1987.
6. Kochamba G, Desrosiers C, Dewar M, et al: The muscle powered dual chamber counterpulsator: rheologically superior implantable cardiac assist device. Ann Thorac Surg. 45:620, 1988.
7. Chiu RC-J, Walsh GL, Dewar ML, et al: Implantable extra-aortic balloon assist

powered by transformed fatigue resistant skeletal muscle. J Thorac Cardiovasc Surg 94:694, 1987.

8. Mannion JD, Velchik M, Alavi A, et al: Blood flow in conditioned and unconditioned latissimus dorsi muscle. J Surg Res 47:332, 1989.

9. Acker MA, Hammond RL, Mannion JD, et al: An autologous biologic pump motor. J Thorac Cardiovasc Surg 92:733, 1986.

10. Acker MA, Hammond RL, Mannion JD, et al: Skeletal muscle as a potential power source for a cardiovascular pump: assessment in vivo. Science 236:324, 1987.

11. Chachques JC, Grandjean P, Schwartz K, et al: Effect of latissimus dorsi dynamic cardiomyoplasty on ventricular function. Circulation (suppl III) 78:203, 1988.

12. Magovern GJ, Heckler FR, Park SB, et al: Paced skeletal muscle for dynamic cardiomyoplasty. Ann Thorac Surg 45:614, 1988.

13. Kusserow BK, Clapp III JF: A small ventricle-type pump for prolonged perfusions: construction and initial studies, including attempts to power a pump biologically with skeletal muscle. Trans Amer Soc Artif Int Organs 10:74–78, 1964.

14. Spotnitz HM, Merker C, Malm JR: Applied physiology of the canine rectus abdominis: force-length curves correlated with functional characteristics of a rectus powered "ventricle"-potential for cardiac assistance. Trans Amer Soc Artif Int Organs 20:747, 1974.

15. Juffe A, Ricoy JR, Marquez J, et al: Cardialization-a new source of energy for circulatory assistance. Vasc Surg 12:10, 1978.

16. Macoviak JA, Stephenson LW, Armenti F, et al: Electrical conditioning of in situ skeletal muscle for replacement of myocardium. J Surg Res 32:429, 1982.

17. Neilson IR, Brister SJ, Khalafalla AS, et al: Left ventricular assistance in dogs using a skeletal muscle powered device for diastolic augmentation. Heart Transplantation 6:343, 1985.

18. Li CM, Hill A, Desrosiers C, et al: A new implantable burst generator for skeletal muscle powered aortic counterpulsation. Trans Am Soc Artif Intern Organs 35:405, 1989.

19. Spiro D, Sonneblick EH: Comparison of the ultrastructural basis of the contractile process in heart and skeletal muscle. Circ Res (suppl II) 14–15:14, 1964.

20. Nakamura K, Glenn WWL: Graft of the diaphragm as a functioning substitute for the myocardium. J Surg Res 4:348, 1964.

21. Mannion JD, Hammond BS, Stephenson LW: Hydraulic pouches of canine latissimus dorsi. J Thorac Cardiovasc Surg 91:534, 1986.

22. Mannion JD, Acker MA, Hammond RL, et al: Power output of skeletal muscle ventricles in circulation: short-term studies. Circulation 76:155, 1986.

23. Kantrowitz A, Wasfie T, Freed PS, et al: Intraaortic balloon pumping, 1967 through 1982: analysis of complications in 733 patients. Am J Cardiol 57:976, 1986.

24. Kantrowitz A, Freed PS, Wasfie T, et al: Permanent cardiac assistance in chronic congestive failure by means of a mechanical auxiliary ventricle. In TMS Chang, Bing-Lin-He (eds): Hemoperfusion and Artificial Organs. Beijing, China Academic Publishers, 1985, pp 159–165.

25. Novoa R, Castle L, Rashidi R, et al: Pacemaker system for chronic diastolic counterpulsation utilizing skeletal muscle as the power source. Pace 12(I):637, 1989.

26. Kantrowitz A: In series temporary and permanent cardiac assistance. In A Kantrowitz (ed): Primers in Artificial Organs, vol 3 J.B. Lippincott Co., Philadelphia, 1988, pp 77–96.

Chapter 22

Polymer Surfaces in Muscle-Powered Cardiac Assist Devices

J. Donald Hill

Arising from two different basic and applied scientific disciplines, conditioned latissimus dorsi muscle technology and mechanical cardiac support systems may now experience a symbiotic relationship in the successful treatment of patients in the late stages of cardiomyopathy. Each technology has the option to be an independent treatment approach. Dynamic cardiomyoplasty does not require a mechanical pumping device, and cardiac assist devices have alternate energy sources. The potential advantages of a combination of these two technologies minimize their individual disadvantages. Dynamic cardiomyoplasty is limited by the size of the heart in Class IV congestive and dilated heart failure patients, and all current energy systems for implanted heart pumps require cumbersome, transcutaneous energy sources that add measurably to the complexity of the system. Joint efforts to make better systems that would sidestep some of the inherent difficulties in each approach are now underway in a number of centers. This unplanned, but timely turn of events, has introduced ideas for new solutions to finally develop a therapy that will make a significant dent in the dismal public health statistics of chronic cardiomyopathy. Before addressing the surface biomaterial issues in heart pumps it would be worthwhile recounting some of the design strategies that have proven successful in medical engineering.

Axioms of Medical Engineering Design

During the genesis of an engineering design effort one always tries to accurately predict performance requirements, while at the same time create a design within defined limitations or conditions (e.g., size, weight, temperature, shape, etc.). The best designed biomaterials are sought to meet a given set of specifications. This is an historically proven way to develop and build technology with a predictable expectation of success. In medical engineering, the "catch-22" to this formula comes in attempting to predict the body's tol-

From *Cardiomyoplasty* edited by Alain Carpentier, MD, PhD, Juan-Carlos Chachques, MD, and Pierre Grandjean, MS © 1991. Futura Publishing Inc., Mount Kisco, NY.

erance and reaction to a device. It is not like building a bridge where one can accurately assess the setting.

Much is understood about how the body reacts to devices, but far more is unknown. Each new approach or biomaterial that is developed carries with it the chance of partial or complete failure due to unanticipated responses by the body. This experience has taught the medical engineering community some practical principles that are referred to in this chapter as "axioms of medical engineering design."

Unity and Completeness of Design

This important guideline must always be kept in mind. The question must be asked, "how can all the desired features be incorporated into the design?" An example of this relating to biomaterials occurred in the development of heart blood pump sacs. Fifteen years ago a flex life of 5 years was the first requirement of blood pumping sacs. When this was accomplished attention was directed to designing a thromboresistant surface. Much progress has been made in this area, but it remains a high priority for improvement. As shown by the work of Gristina,[1] the attraction biomaterials have for bacteria cannot be ignored and a bacteria-resistant function must be designed into new biomaterials. The evolution of biomaterial designs that have to satisfy a broadening array of necessary functions is the driving force in developing new materials for human use. Never proceed with a material that does not meet known or anticipated requirements in the most optimal formulation.

Design Trade-offs Are Always Necessary

A physician will always want the maximum in safety, efficacy, and performance in an implantable device. This usually is not possible. The improvement of one feature is often at the expense of another. The perfect design occasionally occurs when improvement of one feature results in improvement of others. More commonly, one settles for second best, which is minimal losses in any category. In making decisions on these tradeoffs, stringent analysis, forward thinking, and experience are helpful.

Never Try To Second Guess "Mother Nature" On An Important Design Decision

Obtain preliminary information using animal model testing. This is particularly needed when there is little or no basic science knowledge available.

Build In Redundancy Where Possible

In any implantable life support device redundancy is an appealing feature. Due to anatomical constraints that dictate device size and shape and the body's intolerance to unlimited implanted hardware, redundancy often cannot be designed into the device. For example, a blood pumping chamber can seldom be designed with a backup system. Redundancy becomes possible in control and energy systems. Not surprisingly, any weak link in the system could result in total failure. Limits in redundancy mean that quality assurance of any individual components must be near 100%—that's the rule.

Keep It Simple

This is an age-old rule and it is mentioned for one reason. The safety, efficacy, and performance requirements for assist devices are so demanding that complexity and sophistication are necessary. As demonstrated in the aerospace industry, sophistication and complexity brought improvement in performance and safety. This will also be true in cardiac devices. The appropriate wisdom is to avoid introducing unnecessary complexity into a design.

Design for Anticipated Improvements

Where possible, the device should be designed so that future upgrades can be made without requiring total redesign of the device. This is best accomplished by a modular design so that a section can easily be replaced. The time line for a heart pump development program is at least 5 years. During that time there is certain to be improvement in at least one component. Being able to upgrade the device will keep the design current, safe, and effective.

Devices Work Better in Humans Than in Animal Models

Bench testing and animal models are crucial to device development. Since the development of the first heart-lung machine 40 years ago it has become apparent that what worked in animals invariably worked better in humans. This may be related to biological tolerance. Whatever the reason, it is a consistent observation that is welcomed by physicians, engineers, and patients. If at all possible, preliminary clinical studies should be done at an early stage where medically appropriate. Even on a temporary basis, an immense amount of information will be learned, including the effectiveness of the device. Specific characteristics may surface in human use that were not apparent in the bench or animal model.

General Categories of Biomaterials

Usually choice of a biomaterial is dictated by the properties it possesses and how they satisfy the desired function. With varying degrees of success, almost all types of biomaterials have found their way into the body. Polymers are the most common (e.g. fibers, rubbers, and plastics) and are used to fabricate membranes, tubes, fibers, particles, powders, containers or liquid and salt adhesives. Metals are the next most frequently used, predominantly in orthopedic devices. Ceramics and carbons are now being introduced for certain functions appropriate to their special properties. All of the above biomaterials are used in composite use as well.

Specifications for Biomaterials Used in Implantable Blood Pumps

Until now the discussion in this chapter regarding polymers has been in global terms in the composite design of a cardiac device. This section focuses on polymers and their specific role in the surfaces exposed to blood in cardiac devices. What are some of the properties that are essential for polymers to have in this setting? The material must have the necessary physical properties such as strength, elasticity, and flexibility. It must be stable and maintain it's physical properties in vivo over long periods of time. It cannot leach undesirable compounds into the general circulation or induce foreign body reactions (e.g., necrosis,cancer, etc.). It must be able to be purified, modified, and sterilized. It should easily lend itself to a fabrication process. Finally, the properties it has should mimic or substitute for the body's mechanism of keeping blood liquid in the vascular space. What is this mechanism?

Blood Flow and the Endothelium—Why Blood Stays Liquid in the Vascular Space

Blood stays liquid in the vascular space due to a delicate set of balances. Flow continues to dilute activated coagulation products that build up. The endothelium remains nourished so that several functions can be performed (Fig. 1). First, circulation platelets are in an environment where they do not easily stick to damaged endothelium or to each other, or release procoagulant materials into the blood. These functional changes in platelets are produced by the normal low-level production of prostacyclin (PGI_2) by endothelial cells. Second, the endothelium's outer membrane acts as a continuous source of heparinlike material that with antithrombin III can scavenge any activated coagulation factors (such as IX, X, II) to impede the continuing cascade that would otherwise ultimately produce thrombus. Third, the endothelium synthesizes and releases a tissue plasminogen activator (TPA) that can proteolytically cleave fibrin in the area, solubilizing otherwise insoluble thrombus. Fourth, the endothelial membrane has a biochemical mechanism that allows any thrombin that has escaped from the other scavenger systems to destroy other coagulation factors. The intermediaries in these events are proteins C and S, and the "target" to turn off coagulation are probably factors V and VIII. In essence, with normal flow normal endothelium can prevent nonactivated proteins in the blood from making thrombus and promote the destruction of thrombus that has already formed.

WHY BLOOD CLOTS
ON A FOREIGN SURFACE

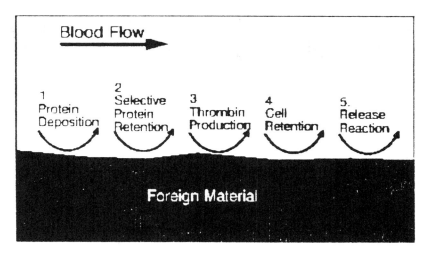

Figure 1. *Protein formation on the foreign surface creates a new surface to which plate-lets and leukocytes adhere, change shape and characteristics, and release materials that promote production of insoluble fibrillar protein that traps red cells.*

Mechanisms of Thrombosis on A Foreign Surface

Once the endothelium is removed, the macroscopic equivalent of the loss of all these vital endothelial functions ensues and there is a strong tendency to thrombose on the replacement surface. Moreover, the several materials that compose a device must be joined creating seams that disturb flow. Even the most biocompatible materials promote platelet retention and activation as well as thrombin generation through the retention and proteolytic cleavage of the coagulation proteins. The lack of endothelial cells that create the walls of these devices can be the "coup de grace"; without these cells, any coagulation that builds up remains because local fibrinolysis is hampered. Understanding the details of how blood is modified by a generic biomaterial is crucial to under-standing continued attempts to optimize the thromboresistance of surface poly-mers in a complex device.

When blood flows through a nonbiological tube, proteins are deposited instantaneously (Fig. 2). Some proteins are retained with or without shape modification or enzymatic alteration. All these proteins create a semistation-ary new biological surface so that the blood is no longer in contact with the polymer that initiated these reactions. Enzymatic reactions produce both small molecular weight peptide fragments and other enzymes. These enzymes change other blood-derived proteins into enzymes active in the promotion and eventual dissolution of fibrin. The production of complement and kinin components also

WHY BLOOD STAYS LIQUID
IN A BLOOD VESSEL

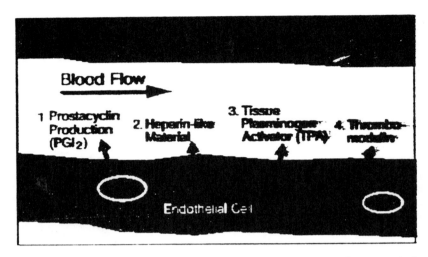

Figure 2. *Blood stays liquid in the vascular space due to flow and enzymatic function of the normal endothelium.*

occur. Independently but simultaneously, platelets and leukocytes adhere to the new protein layer, change their membranes, and release a wide variety of materials, some of which promote production of an insoluble fibrillar protein matrix that traps red cells.

In this example, the polymeric material has replaced the normal endothelium. Therefore, the absence of the endothelial cell, and thus one source for thrombolysis, is lost in the microenvironment (Fig. 2). Normally, blood stays liquid in the vascular space, not only due to flow, but because the dominant enzymatic function of the unaltered endothelium is to lyse thrombi. Only normal endothelium can: (1) generate specific prostaglandins to impede platelet retention and the release reaction; (2) release tissue plasminogen activator (TPA) that triggers the production of fibrinolytic enzymes and ultimately thrombus dissolution; (3) modify thrombin from a prothrombotic enzyme to one that increases plasmin production; and (4) express heparin on their surface that retain and activate antithrombin III to break down the coagulation enzymes. Many of the reactions continue long after the initiation of thrombosis not only propagating the thrombus but modifying it in many ways.

The endothelial area of the body's vascular space is large and is now recognized to have the sophisticated biological functions normally associated with a specialized organ. The endothelium functions as an endocrine organ but cannot by itself inhibit thrombosis. There must be flow and no area of stasis.

For example, unaltered fibrinogen or fragments leave the surface within minutes, and retained platelets also re-enter the flowing blood within hours.

Cross-linking of the fibrin and cell death in the retained material also occurs. Some of these reactions, no doubt, contribute to changes in the polymeric vessel that is seen weeks to months later, although the specific reactions producing these clinical events have not been identified. No knowledge exists concerning what triggers a new round of thromboembolism weeks or months later, although the specific reactions producing these clinical events have not been identified. One of these events, delayed embolism from thrombus on a device, needs to be avoided at all costs.

Types of Cardiac Support Devices

Device complexity is linked to the level of mechanical cardiac support desired. For each of these devices the latissimus dorsi muscle could be an attractive internal chronic energy source to power a cardiac device. Three general types of devices can be considered: counterpulsation devices inside, parallel to, or part of the thoracic aorta; myocardial wall or intracavitary displacement devices; or prosthetic ventricles that provide total cardiac output requirements. The latter can be implanted orthotopically, in which case the native heart is removed and replaced by left and right prosthetic ventricles; or heterotopically, where the devices are attached to the retained native heart by way of large bore cannulae either unilaterally or bilaterally. Prosthetic ventricles could be entirely mechanical, receiving energy from the in situ latissimus dorsi muscle or by transposing the muscle to surround the pumping device. All of these devices have significant blood contact surfaces. Balloon and displacement devices, which can also derive their power from the latissimus dorsi muscle, have the least total blood contact surface with the most homogeneous biomaterial surface seen by the blood. Prosthetic ventricles, however, have the largest blood contacting surface and present in a variety of shapes and compositions. Using the Thoratec prosthetic pump (Berkeley, CA) as an example, the following section traces the path the blood takes and the unfamiliar surfaces it will encounter as it traverses the device.

Surfaces Blood Encounters Traversing A Blood Pump

The blood first encounters the polyurethane external and internal surface of the inlet cannula in the left ventricular apex or the left atrium. The junction between the tissue and the external surface of the cannula is also located in these sites. As the blood traverses down the cannula to the inlet valve, there are two seams that signify both change in surface and a ledge (microscopic though it may be): the cannula connector seam and the connector valve seam. Under the valve (a major foreign surface because of its associated flow turbulence) there is an additional seam between it and the polyurethane sac. Beyond the sac there are the same potential thrombotic sites in the outflow conduit plus the polyurethane cannula-Dacron graft junction and finally the Dacron graft to the pulmonary artery or aortic anastomosis. Clearly, there are many sources for thrombus formation and not only the sac can be viewed as the cause. All prosthetic ventricles have these sites to a greater or lesser degree. In contemplating the final design of a surface, all of these factors must be considered. The theoretical goal is to have one continuous antithrombogenic surface along a physiological blood flow path fabricated of material that has a 5-year (200 million cycle) flex life. An antibacterial surface would be an additionally welcomed feature particularly in light of the increased information linking infection to thromboembolism. A single mold of the blood path through the device as noted above would be desirable for medical and economic reasons, but is not yet possible. At present, keeping the blood contact components to a minimum or creating a continuous polymer coat over the blood contact surface is a realistic alternative. As final specifications, the device must be able to be scaled up or down in size, have near perfect quality assurance, and be manufactured at reasonable cost.

There are components of a heart pump that do not come in contact with blood but are adjacent to other body tissues and should be inert if possible. These include the compliance chamber, energy converter, control system, internal battery, and transcutaneous energy system. The last item and possibly some of the other items might not be necessary if the latissimus dorsi muscle's energy can be harnessed.

Types of Blood Compatible Surfaces for Heart Pumps

Twenty years ago, because of a wide variety of prosthetic device needs in cardiovascular surgery, work on usable blood compatible biomaterials began in earnest. Over time a number of excellent blood compatible surfaces have evolved. In the prosthetic heart pump field, most of the concentration on nonthrombogenic surfaces is focused on the blood sac despite the knowledge that thromboembolic material can arise from a number of sites in the device. This is understandable since the sac is and has been considered the core of the device with the largest blood surface contact area and the requirement to flex 40 million times per year. The imperfections of the blood sac had to be solved first so that attention could be directed to other sites.

Before describing some of the surfaces that have been successfully used in devices it is worthwhile to reflect on another ingredient that contributes to success; the art and craft of polymer fabrication. The proper design and biomaterials are critical but experience and know-how are equally important. Handling these materials can be difficult and often taken for granted by less experienced people until transfer of technology is followed by a protracted period of trial, error, and a learning curve until a new group masters the fabrication. In addition, this fabrication must be reproducible time after time with perfect quality control.

Smooth Polyurethane

Fabricating polymer sacs with smooth surfaces was the first approach used in developing antithrombogenic surfaces. Before any significant progress was made, it was recognized that the flex life of most of these polymers was no more than 3 months. In the mid 1970s Dupont (Wilmington, Delaware) developed a segmented polyurethane called Biomer® for use in the garment industry. They licensed this material to Ethicon (Somerville, NJ) for medical applications. Biomer® has bulk characteristics that are resistant to flex ware and has proven to be a valuable biomaterial in medical technology. By chance, the surface of Biomer® proved to be surprisingly antithrombogenic and in combination with its long flex life became the first successful bladder to be used in heart pumps. Examining the formulation of Biomer® reveals that it contains a number of impurities that can show up on the surface of a completed sac. These impurities can be removed and result in improved blood compatibility. Examples of these improved segmented polyurethanes are Angiothane®and Thermothane®. The requirement for a long flex life and a blood compatible surface have been addressed separately with Thoratec's (Berkeley, CA) BSP— 215M smooth segmented polyurethane. BSP 215M is composed of a purified segmented polyurethane to give it a long flex life and is then mixed with a co-polymer. The co-polymer migrates to the surface during the fabrication process providing improved blood compatible characteristics. It has proven to be better than purified Biomer® in controlled studies. The amphipathic structure of the surface being neither hydrophobic nor hydrophillic adjusts to its environment. This material is now in clinical use in the Thoratec prosthetic ventricle.

Further improvements in smooth polyurethane bladders will include substances to retard infection and possibly biologically active compounds on the surface that mimic the functions of the endothelium.

Textured Blood Surface Interface

In the mid-1960s early investigations using smooth polymer surfaces were not successful. There was a lack of basic science knowledge in choosing the most appropriate chemical surface, and investigations of different biomaterials largely were done by a trial and error approach. Creating an endothelialized surface on a foreign material was an attractive idea, and textured surfaces were developed for that specific purpose. A smooth adherent clot will develop on a textured surface following contact with blood. The initial premise was that this thrombus over time would become a continuous endothelial surface. What eventually evolved was more of a pseudoendothelial surface, but it has proven to be very antithrombogenic. Initially the textured surfaces were fabricated by evenly attaching polyester fibers to the surface of a polymer bladder. Polyurethane fibers are now also used to produce textured surfaces. A more recent development is the integration of the textured surface directly into the sac by producing excavations that are formed through a solution-casting process. All of these textured surfaces have enviable records in a long history of laboratory experiments. Their antithrombogenic properties are well established. They have been used successfully clinically over relatively short periods of time. One lingering apprehension exists when long-term use in humans is anticipated. In animal laboratory experiments in which the animal model was usually in a growth stage of its development, calcification of the pseudoendothelium was observed. Whether this will manifest itself in adult patients who are not in a growth phase is unknown.

A further development in textured endothelial surfaces is the use of seeding techniques to improve the quality and extent of the endothelial growth. These methods of mimicking "mother nature" will continue to have an important role in the future.

Biolized Surfaces

A biolized surface is one treated with gelatin,[3-6] which renders it very compatible with blood. The gelatin biological surface is passive in nature. Despite its success it has not been widely adapted by other groups partly because there is a large element of art and craft in its fabrication.

Biologically Active Surface

Basic science investigations on blood and endothelium increasingly point to the fact that the physiological basis of coagulation resides mainly in the blood, whereas the vascular endothelium plays the predominant role in keeping the blood in a liquid state. This information has led investigators to develop biologically active surfaces that will mimic the function of the endothelium. As long as 15–20 years ago heparin ionically bonded to a foreign surface was used with moderate success to prevent clotting, but it could not be relied upon and was not durable. Olson and coworkers at the Karolinska Institute in Stockholm, Sweden, dramatically changed this by covalently bonding heparin to a foreign surface with end-point attachment.[7] Antithrombin III adheres to the heparin on the surface and effectively inhibits thrombin. This covalently bonded heparin can be applied to a variety of surfaces having a variety of shapes and contours. Once again, the flow patterns in these devices must avoid stagnant flow or thrombosis can occur. Covalently bonded heparin is chemically attached to the surface and therefore is not easily removed. This feature has given this material considerable durability to maintain its antithrombogenic properties. There is now considerable experience in performing clinical ECMO without heparin and without evidence of thrombosis or consumption of coagulation factors.[8,9] This material has not been used on the sacs of prosthetic hearts, but there is no reason why it would not be successful.

Protein-Specific Adsorbing Surface

This method was developed by Eberhart and his group in Dallas.[10] They developed a chemically modified silicon rubber surface that attracts albumin. The albumin in turn represents a friendly, if not chemically active surface, to the blood flowing over it. The coagulation cascade is not stimulated and the surface remains thrombus-free. This technology has not been clinically evaluated but has great promise as a valuable addition to antithrombogenic surfaces.

Systemic Anticoagulation to Inhibit Surface Thrombosis of Blood-Contacting Devices

This is an indirect means of altering the risk of thrombosis on a device. The continued need to employ this approach emphasizes the continuing failure to develop a long-lasting and effective antithrombogenic surface.

The cornerstone of this approach is to use Coumadin, heparin, and antiplatelet drugs in various combinations. Once systemic anticoagulation is added to the regimen to inhibit thrombosis bleeding becomes a risk.

Detecting Thrombosis in Implanted Blood Pumps

The understanding of how thrombus forms has led to a number of advances in models to detect and quantitate thrombus on a device. Each method has advantages and limitations. Anatomical visualization of the thrombus on the device has been accomplished by radiographic and ultrasound techniques. Sequential ultrasound has the advantage of being noninvasive and easily repeated, but it only semiquantitatively assesses thrombosis on a device. Device movement—universal to a pump attached to the heart—only diminishes the sensitivity more. Use of radionuclide tagging of native blood components that participate to form the thrombus has been impractical. Platelets tagged with [111]Indium and fibrogen labeled with radionuclide iodine or technetium have been qualitative measurements only.

Methods to assess accelerated turnover of these components of the blood to estimate thrombogenesis have also been suboptimal. In animal models, the specificity of these tests has been confounded by the effects of surgery and infection on the blood elements. In humans, more confounding variables exist such as the effect of drugs and other therapeutic interventions.

Sequential blood tests to assess the in vivo platelet release reaction (using B-thromboglobulin and platelet factor IV); in vivo thrombin transformation of fibrinogen (using fibrinopeptide A); and depression of antithrombin III levels (implying accelerated removal when bound to activated coagulation factors) currently are being evaluated.

Conclusion

There are no perfect blood compatible surfaces. The ones that are available are acceptable for clinical application and are being used with excellent results. For years the difficulty in fabricating these surfaces has been underestimated. Surgeons, being optimists, have always thought the solution was nearly in site, but progress is slow. The recognition of the vital role that basic science inquiries have played in the formulation of surfaces has only been truly appreciated in the last decade. Future improvements will come one at a time along with better predictability of their special in vivo performance. Now there is much to be optimistic about.

References

1. Gristina AG, Dobbins JJ, Giammara B, et al: Biomaterial centered sepsis and the total artificial heart: microbial adhesion vs tissue integration. JAMA 259:870, 1988.
2. Farrar DJ, Litwak P, Lawson JH, et al: In vivo evaluations of a new thromboresistant polyurethane for artificial heart blood pumps. J Thor Cardiovasc Surg 95:191, 1988.
3. Emoto H, Murabayashi S, Kambic HE, et al: Plasma protein and gelatin surface interactions: kinetics of protein adsorption. Trans Am Soc Artif Intern Organs 33:606, 1987.
4. Kambic H, Murabayashi S, Jacobs G, et al: Cardiac prostheses: toward permanent implantation. Cleve Clin Quart 51:105, 1984.
5. Kambic H, Myrabayashi S, Harasaki H, et al: Composite polymeric materials: evaluation of crosslinked gel protein surfaces. Proc Intl Soc Artif Organs 3:203, 1979.
6. Kambic H, Murabayashi S, Harasaki H, et al: Characterization of protein coating for functional cardiac prosthesis. Proc Intl Soc Artif Organs 5:526, 1981.
7. Larsson R, Larm O, Olsson P: The search for thromboresistance using immobilized heparin. In "Blood Contact with Natural and Artificial Surfaces" N.Y. Acad Sciences 516:102, 1987.
8. Mottaghy K, et al: Heparin free long term extracorporeal circulation using bioactive surfaces. Trans Am Soc Artif Intern Organs 1989.
9. Peters J: Extracorporeal CO2 removal with a heparin coated artificial lung. Intens Care Med 14:578, 1988.
10. Eberhart RC, Munro MS, Frautschi JR, et al: Influence of indigenous albumin binding on blood material interactions. In "Blood Contact with Natural and Artificial Surfaces" N.Y. Acad. Sciences 516:78, 1987.

Part IV
Conclusion

Chapter 23

Conclusion: From Results to Indications

Alain Carpentier

At the end of this book, it seems desirable to answer the question that is on everyone's mind: What is the place of dynamic cardiomyoplasty in the armamentarium of cardiac surgery? This question has two answers: one present and one future. At the present time, the persistent uncertainties and limitations underscored in the various chapters of this book show that this operation is still in its development phase. For the future, it is clear that experimental and clinical efficiency shows great promise. The fact that continuous fatigueless contraction of a skeletal muscle at the frequency of the heart has been obtained for periods of more than five years in the human is in itself remarkable. The fact that most patients were functionally improved with a significant increase in cardiac output and ejection fraction in some of them is encouraging. Finally, the fact that similar results have been obtained by various physicians throughout the world, provided that they had access to burst train generators, demonstrates that the operation is feasible.

But efficiency and feasibility are only two of the many requirements that are necessary to transform an operation into a surgical tool. Reliability is also important and this has not been achieved thus far. The variability of the results obtained seems to be linked in part to multiple technical details and in part to the heterogenicity of the patients operated on. Any new operation faces such shortcomings in its developmental phase. Continuous improvements in technique and selection of patients should serve to increase reliability. Also disappointing is the fact that the mechanism of this operation remains to be elucidated. The transmission of the muscle contraction to the underlying cardiac tissue probably does not play a major role. Other factors such as stabilization of the ventricular wall during systole, upper displacement of the heart during muscular contraction, and possible cross revascularization also must be considered and need further evaluation.

Current indications must stem from current results. These were a matter of heated discussion and strong controversy during the round table entitled "From Results to Indications," which took place during the first meeting on Dynamic Cardiomyoplasty in Paris in 1989. I could not find a better answer

From *Cardiomyoplasty* edited by Alain Carpentier, MD, PhD, Juan-Carlos Chachques, MD, and Pierre Grandjean, MS © 1991. Futura Publishing Inc., Mount Kisco, NY.

to the crucial question of indications than publishing the report of this round table, which was so efficiently chaired by Dr. Wellens.

Alain Carpentier, MD, PhD

From Results to Indications

WELLENS (Chairman):   As of June, 1989 fifty plus patients had cardiomyoplasty with a follow-up extending over 4 years in Carpentier's series. Is there a critical heart size where we can expect that the power developed by the latissimus dorsi will be insufficient to move that heart inward? That information would be of help to recognize patients that will probably not benefit from the procedure.

SALMONS: Yes is the answer, there must be. The fully transformed muscle has a maximum power of about 40 watts per gram if you can arrange that the muscle is contracting at the "peak" of the curve. Forty watts per gram is exactly the same for the power developed by a normal heart during systole. There is enough power, but you have to load the muscle under the right conditions. If the load is very great you can develop force in the muscle, but the muscle is unable to contract and so you don't get any power. It is much more difficult to try to calculate what the diameter can be because you are wrapping the muscle around another muscle, the cardiac wall. You do not know what the transfer of pressure is across that cardiac wall. If the cardiac wall was made of metal, the pressure inside the chamber would not be transferred at all to the skeletal muscle. Now, at some lesser stage there is some compliance, which will vary from patient to patient. So it is extremely difficult to calculate, but one would predict, certainly with a very large heart, that the muscle is not helping by squeezing the heart but in some other fashion. In many people's experience it seems that there is not a lot of difference between single pulse and burst stimulation. And yet, there are important differences in terms of skeletal muscle contraction between those two. Maybe that is an indication that it is not actual contraction that is doing the benefit to the patient.

WELLENS: One of the things I missed this morning was a discussion on the relation between heart size and improvement or lack of improvement. I would like to call upon a few of the people that presented data this morning to hear their opinion. Dr. Moreira, would you like to comment on the relation between size and results?

MOREIRA: Our patients showed a correlation between the size of the heart and the results obtained after cardiomyoplasty. In patients in whom we had the opportunity to wrap the entire heart, we observed a great increase in the ejection fraction of both ventricles. Patients that had a major cardiac enlargement, showed only small benefit.

WELLENS: Dr. Magovern, are you going to reject people when the diameter of the right and left ventricles taken together is 15 cm or more?

MAGOVERN: Perhaps I am a little bit critical since I do not know how this operation works. My own feeling is that with the anterior wrap, as we see it in the echo and other studies, posteriorly the heart becomes adherent. If a muscle is pulling this way and it can raise the heart up as you see it when you first apply it, it simply lifts it up. If it can't lift it up, then it is going to compress it down. It works very much as external compression of the heart on the anterior and anterolateral chest wall. So that's why I am not certain that dimension per se and how much you wrap is totally critical. I think it is a form of external compression, only it is done internally, particularly with the anterior wrap. Now, I think probably if you have a very dilated cardiomyopathy and you cannot get a complete wrap, that might be different.

WELLENS: Prof. Carpentier, what is the Broussais experience concerning the relation between effect of cardiomyoplasty and size of the heart?

CARPENTIER: It would be preferable to talk about ventricular volumes rather than heart size. As you know, it is not only the pressure within these ventricles which counteract skeletal muscle contraction but namely the tension on the ventricular wall. This tension, given by the Laplace's law, is proportional to the pressure and to the radius of the ventricle. The larger the radius the higher the tension and therefore the more difficult for the muscle to squeeze the heart. Anyone who has had the occasion of practicing cardiac massage on dilated hearts has been able to feel this. In addition, large ventricles are difficult to wrap completely. For these two reasons, very large ventricles are a contra-indication to cardiomyoplasty unless their size is reduced to reasonable dimensions in the same time a cardiomyoplasty is performed.

WELLENS: Talking about indications, you can also approach it from the other end and talk about contraindications. The Broussais experience mentioned three situations, and I would like to discuss them separately.
    Valve pathology, severe arrhythmias, and pulmonary insufficiency were considered to be contraindications. Large hearts usually have mitral valve incompetence and tricuspid incompetence. How much incompetence are we going to accept? How much is Dr. Moreira accepting?

MOREIRA: We only avoid patients with a high degree of mitral regurgitation. We accept patients with light or moderate mitral regurgitation. Preferably we have to select patients with only low degrees of mitral regurgitation. Patients with a moderate degree of mitral incompetence may also be submitted to cardiomyoplasty, but they may need a valvular reconstruction or replacement in the future.

WELLENS: Dr. Carpentier and Dr. Mihaileanu, you gave us the impression that while in the past you combined cardiomyoplasty with mitral valve surgery, you are no longer doing this. Is that true?

MIHAILEANU: In moderate or even mild mitral insufficiency, cardiomyoplasty does not affect afterload. It increases contractility and therefore increases mitral insufficiency. In the presence of moderate mitral insufficiency, unless repair or replacement is done, there is no good indication for cardio-myoplasty.

WELLENS: Are you accepting moderate mitral incompetence without ele-vation of right-sided pressures?

MIHAILEANU: Very moderate, yes.

WELLENS: During the last year, what percentage of patients presented to you were accepted for cardiomyoplasty?

MIHAILEANU: During the last 2-year period, where as you have seen the operative mortality has been reduced less than 10% we, maybe, rejected 30% of the patients.

WELLENS: What do you mean by maybe?

MIHAILEANU: I don't have the exact percentages.

WELLENS: But that's a very important point. Prof. Carpentier, what is your impression?

CARPENTIER: It is difficult for Dr. Mihaileanu to answer your question be-cause during the development phase of such a new operation, the indications vary considerably as the experience grows. Practically speaking, whenever a patient is referred to us for an end-stage cardiac disease requiring some sort of cardiac support, we first determine whether a cardiac transplantation is indicated. Whenever a cardiac transplantation is contraindicated—or the pa-tient refuses this alternative—we discuss whether a cardiomyoplasty is pos-sible with a reasonable chance of success. A reasonable chance of success exists when the heart still has a "myocardial reserve" i.e., an acceptable contractility of the base of the ventricles and when none of the following contraindications is present:

1. Significant mitral valve insufficiency is a contraindication because it does not make sense to me to increase the regurgitation by increasing ventricular contraction. Of course, we could repair or replace the mitral valve, but one has to weigh the risk of this additional procedure. I think it is too early to take this risk because our main objective is to determine whether this operation works rather than to evaluate its indications whenever associated valvular diseases are present.
2. Severe arrhythmias are also a contraindication although we have had two patients whose arrhythmia improved after cardiomyoplasty. But arrhythmia makes it more difficult to synchronize the myostimulator.
3. Severely impaired pulmonary function is also a contraindication be-cause the thoracotomy and the muscle inside the chest worsen it.
4. Finally, I don't like to operate on patients with a critical stenosis of a coronary artery that cannot be bypassed because of diffuse lesions. These patients have a high risk of massive myocardial infarction in the following months or years and the cardiomyoplasty is not going to prevent this risk.

Let me repeat that large ventricles and aneurysms are not a contraindication provided that their size is reduced. Dr. Wellens, I don't want to elude your question on the proportion of patients we have rejected, but it has varied so much in this past 2 years that any number would have no statistical value.

WELLENS: Any comments from other members of the panel or questions from the floor?

QUESTION FROM THE AUDIENCE: Dr. Magovern, some of your patients showed obvious clinical improvement with stimulation in spite of any change in ventricular systolic function as assessed by invasive measurements or echocardiography. Do you have any explanation concerning this discrepancy and what about the diastolic function in these patients?

MAGOVERN: I think that noninvasive testing is very subjective. The patient knows when you are turning the pacer on and off. We try to avoid telling them, but they can feel the muscle when it is working. So you get a subjective degree of cooperation. As I told you yesterday, in the ones that are improved, their ejection fraction does not necessarily change a great deal but the configuration of the ventricle apparently does, and we see stability of the septum without the paradoxical motion. I think that septal stability plus configuration of the ventricle perhaps accounts for the improvement in cardiac output.

SALMONS: A lot of people are basing a part of their assessment on Doppler and echocardiography. I wonder how reliable this technique is in this situation because the heart is actually being lifted during the contraction of the muscle. You could simply be looking at a change in cross section as the heart passes through the beam of the ultrasound. Perhaps people could comment on that.

WELLENS: It is certainly striking to see the discrepancy between the outcome of Doppler, echo, or nuclear techniques and the clinical picture. Possibly, exercise testing can give us a better idea about functional improvement.

MOREIRA: I'd like to comment about indications for cardiomyoplasty. I agree with Dr. Carpentier, when he talked about the contraindication of mitral regurgitation and very large ventricles. On the other hand, when we look for arrhythmias, the majority of the patients with this kind of disease also have a high incidence of arrhythmias. I think that this is not an important limitation. We can observe a good synchronization between the muscle and the heart signal and we can avoid major problems because of arrhythmias. If you consider arrhythmias as a contraindication we only have the possibility to help a small portion of patients with a dilated cardiomyopathy.

CARPENTIER: I did not say arrhythmias but "severe arrhythmias" and particularly ventricular extrasystole or episodes of ventricular tachycardia. Again, our problem in these days is not to enlarge the indications, but to evaluate the efficiency of this operation under the best scientific conditions. Introducing too many variables will make it more difficult to judge its efficiency. Let us first select pure, severe myocardial insufficiency with no associated lesions. There are enough patients of this type.

WELLENS: For example . . .

CARPENTIER: For example, patients suffering from ischemic heart disease with diffuse coronary artery disease but well developed collateral circulation and no critical coronary artery stenosis, patients with dilated cardiomyopathy without valve incompetence and patients with giant left ventricular aneurysm and poor ventricular function of the remaining myocardium without severe arrhythmias.

As far as Dr. Salmons question regarding the evaluation of the efficiency of the operation and a potential misinterpretation resulting from the lifting of the heart during muscular contraction, Dr. Levy may shed some light on this question.

LEVY: Tomography with multiple slices may overcome this problem. Here is for example a tomography of Madame P, who had a cardiomyoplasty following removal of a myocardial tumor by Dr. Carpentier 4 years ago. As you can see, we can evaluate the regional wall motion and calculate the local ejection fraction from apex to base. In the case of this patient the calculated ejection fraction is about 40 to 50% at the apex and at the base. Another Dr. Carpentier's patient, Mrs. D, had a dilated cardiomyopathy. The scans before the operation showed the right ventricle to be enlarged with a global akinesis. Ejection fraction near the apex was calculated between 10 to 20% and near the base about 40%. After operation, the right ventricle was less enlarged and the left ventricle more kinetic without akinetic areas. Ejection fraction near the apex was 30% but remained almost the same, i.e., 35% to 40% at the base. This method is a tomo-acquisition. We can reconstruct 12 slices from apex to base and thus eliminate errors resulting from the motion of the heart under the effect of the muscle contraction.

WELLENS: A very important question that we should address is the functional classification of the patient. Most of us are looking for patients in Class −IV or III+, but I had the impression that the patient who was operated yesterday was a little less than Class 3, and I was just wondering whether Broussais is moving a little bit away from the strict criterium they had before that the patient should be in Class IV or III+.

CARPENTIER: I do agree that the patient I operated on yesterday may have seemed to you a borderline indication since he was in functional Class III at the time of the operation. However, his cardiologist insisted that a cardiomyoplasty be done because his condition worsened recently. He had had several episodes of pulmonary edema that were more and more difficult to control. The myocardial biopsy showed an extensive myocardial fibrosis. The only alternative would have been a cardiac transplantation at a later stage, but the patient refused this alternative. You probably have been more satisfied with the condition of the second patient I operated on today. He was in functional Class IV but not beyond the possibility of surgery since he still had some contractility of the base of the left ventricle. In general, I consider that the best indications today are what I call "intermittent Class IV" patients, i.e., patients having had one or two episodes of pulmonary edema in spite of adequate medical treatment and diet, but who still have a "myocardial reserve," allowing them to have a reduced, but still acceptable physical activity between the episodes of decompensation.

WELLENS: That is quite clear as far as the functional classification is concerned. We have seen that there is time needed for the transposed muscle to get good contact with the heart. The time interval usually accepted between the operation and the start of the adaptation process is 2 weeks. Is that under all circumstances the correct time? What factors determine the time interval between the operation and the first pacing attempt?

MAGOVERN: I think you can start pacing earlier, but only to the degree that you are going to convert the muscle, not in terms of increasing contractility. If you do that too early you just rip the muscle off the heart. I believe that conversion can be started earlier: after about 10 days.

MIHAILEANU: You can start conversion 5 to 6 days earlier, but it takes at least 6 weeks before you get the full hemodynamic effect, so it would not be a great benefit. The problem is to go through these difficult weeks after surgery, because we do not have any hemodynamic benefit of the cardiomyoplasty at that time.

MOREIRA: I agree with these ideas. I think that the pacing delay is important and while it may be shorter it should not compromise the effect. I would like to comment that the real improvement using Carpentier's progressive sequential stimulation protocol is observed only after the first month of stimulation. Therefore, we have to support the patient with medications during one month and a half, without great benefit from the wrapped muscle.

CARPENTIER: Dr. Moreira is right and I will go even further. The benefit you can get from the operation does not show up clearly before 3 months and continues to increase up to 6 months and even 1 year. Two patients told me that they continued to improve all along the whole year following their operation.

WELLENS: The conclusion is that a period in between 10 to 18 days should pass before pacing can be started and that it takes 6 months to 1 year to evaluate the benefit of the operation.

METRAS: I have a question for the panel. Now that you are becoming more confident about the efficiency of this operation: how would you make your choice between a cardiac transplant and cardiomyoplasty?

MAGOVERN: That is a very hypothetical situation. At this point, if the patient is really bad enough to need a heart transplantation, we would not advise a muscle wrap. But, because of the scarcity of organs in the United States, I would prefer to go ahead with the muscle wrap in a patient in their forties because I do not think that will contraindicate subsequent transplantation. I think we will be using it and we are using it for that indication. You have to be in Class VI and in the hospital on dopamine, etc. to get a transplant today in the U.S.

WELLENS: Where do you draw the line, Professor Carpentier?

CARPENTIER: I do not draw any line. This is an experimental technique or, more exactly, a technique still in its experimental phase so that if a line is to be drawn, it is a dotted line! The policy we have had at Broussais has been influenced strongly by ethical considerations. We have reserved this operation to those patients having a contraindication, whether clinical, social, or psychological, to heart transplantation. But as Dr. Magovern pointed out, the fact that in the U.S. a cardiac transplant candidate is awaiting the last term of his disease to get, or not to get, a heart makes it worth it to propose cardiomyoplasty as an alternative to cardiac transplantation. The more so that there is still a possibility to do a cardiac transplantation later. However, I would recommend that cardiomyoplasty be done at an earlier stage whenever possible.

QUESTION FROM THE AUDIENCE: I am a little bit unhappy, perhaps similar to the others, not to see a uniform good result from this operation with improvement of cardiac function. We have seen different results from different parts of the world and I think it probably all comes to one thing: we are not timing the muscle contraction correctly and I think that this is probably similar to cardiac massage. There is no point in getting that muscle to contract at the time of the isometric contraction of the heart if you have a largely dilated heart because of a large volume. Important, I think is to squeeze that muscle during the isotonic contraction of the left ventricle. Probably the thing you need is a Millar catheter in the left ventricle to tell you what is the maximum point of Dp/Dt which immediately tells you what is the isotonic contraction. As long as you do not time the contraction and you do not convince this audience that the ejection fraction or the cardiac output goes up by a certain percentage, I think that the fight over who is going to benefit from the operation will continue.

WELLENS: Timing of the contraction is a very important point but the pacing devices that are available allow you to change the time of contraction of the latissimus dorsi. That has to be done on a individualized basis because the correct time of contraction varies from patient to patient.

We have been listening to very interesting discussions concerning a technique which is still in an investigational state. Many questions will have to be answered and I would like to suggest to start an international registry on cardiomyoplasty. There are already many international registries, as for electrical ablation in patients with arrhythmias, the long QT-syndrome, PTCA, etc., such an approach is very important to help us to obtain more definite conclusions as to indications for this new and innovative method which may help patients with poor pump function.

I would like to thank the members of the panel and give the microphone back to Professor Carpentier.

CARPENTIER CLOSING: Thank you Dr. Wellens for having chaired this stimulating session. I wish to make it clear that we have not been trying to convince anyone, we have just been trying to evaluate a new operation as much as we could. It is no surprise to me that there are still some obscure points, that improvements are necessary, and that the indications are not as well defined as we would like! It is the fate of any new medical technique. It is no surprise either that results varied from one group to another since there were variations in the application of the technique in part due to the limited availability of the myostimulator. The surprise rather comes from the fact that this operation has proven to remain effective in numerous cases after several years even though we are not able to understand the exact mechanism by which it worked and this, in itself, is the most important message of this meeting. Of course, improvements are mandatory: more precise clinical indications, more efficient surgical technique, and more rigorous postoperative evaluation are the aims we must persue in the forthcoming years. A matter of discussion for the next meeting in two years.

ADDENDUM

The following information became available at the time of publication. To provide the most up-to-date information, the publisher has chosen to include the following addendum.

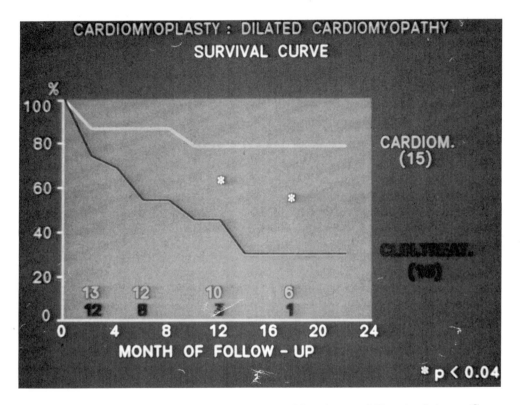

The above figure was received from Dr. F. Moreira and Dr. A. Jatene (Sao Paulo, Brazil). It shows the 2-year survival in two series of patients matched in terms of functional class and disability. One group was treated medically while the other underwent a cardiomyoplasty. There was a striking difference in the mortality rates at 2 years between these two series. This significant difference demonstrates that in addition to the significant functional benefit underlined in this book, this operation seems to be able to stabilize the underlying disease process, probably by interrupting the vicious cycle of progressive dilatation and by reinforcing the residual myocardial contraction, thus improving its efficiency.

AC

Index